Viruses and Colds
The Modern Plague

# Viruses and Colds

## THE MODERN PLAGUE

John M. Adams, M.D., Ph.D.

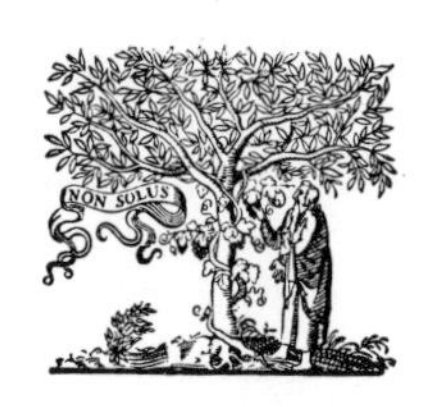


New York

American Elsevier Publishing Company

*Sole Distributors for Great Britain*
Elsevier Publishing Company, Ltd.
Rippleside Commercial Estate
Barking, Essex, England

*Sole Distributors for the Continent of Europe*
Elsevier Publishing Company
335 Jan Van Galenstraat, P.O. Box 211
Amsterdam, The Netherlands

*Library of Congress Catalog Card Number 67–17937*



*Manufactured in The United States of America*

# Contents

# Preface

I intend to tell you the facts, as we know them today, about the most common diseases of mankind. These illnesses in their milder forms are called "colds"; in their more serious forms they are pneumonia, heart disease, or brain fever (encephalitis). The same viruses that cause colds may infect us without our knowledge, and occasionally they may cause overwhelming illness and death. The events concerned with the discovery of the causes, and the brilliant discoverers of them, make thrilling stories, which have been vividly told in many places. I shall take the opportunity throughout this book to refer briefly to them. My principal aim, however, will be to focus on the newer knowledge of these common illnesses and the known causes of many of them, and to discuss a few diseases not caused by viruses but closely resembling those that are. To understand viruses, our tiniest enemies, it is necessary to know where they live and multiply, how they spread among us causing disease, and the best means of counterattack. This is the vital message of this book.

Many viruses live with us. For example, adenoviruses cause tonsillitis and pneumonia, and herpes viruses cause "cold sores" and rarely serious eye disease and encephalitis. Some viruses appear in epidemics and are known to be spread by coughing and sneezing. Influenza and measles are prime examples. Direct means of attack against influenza is in the research laboratory, and vaccines are now safe and effective.

Poliomyelitis, dreaded for a hundred years, can now be controlled through vaccines. Poliovirus causes mild "summer colds" or no illness and gives protection probably for life against the particular type of virus. There are three known types, all of which are included in the vaccines. Other viruses in the same group as polio may rarely cause paralysis. They are also responsible for coldlike illnesses and occasionally involve the brain with a disease called encephalitis. These virus diseases are known as Coxsackie and ECHO infections. Measles is a hard cold with a rash; the aftereffects are serious. The new vaccines are highly effective.

The discovery of the *cause* of a disease represents a great step forward in the battle against our common foe, but many years may be required before protective vaccines or other weapons of attack are available. For example, the virus of polio was discovered in 1908 by Karl Landsteiner, but it was only after it was found to grow in tissue cell cultures that vaccines were developed, nearly fifty years later. Yellow fever was identified as a virus disease at the turn of the century by Walter Reed, and it was again fifty years before Max Theiler demonstrated an effective vaccine. No quick solution for the prevention of colds should be expected, but ways and means are available and the problem is solvable.

The task of presenting the newly acquired truths is not an easy one. This story is told in language that is, hopefully, understandable to all. At a recent National Symposium on "Communications and Medical Research," Dr. Sidney Farber stated: "May I say at once that the public has the right to be informed concerning developments in medical research, particularly with reference to the *causation, prevention* and *treatment* of disease, and the interpretation of discoveries in the laboratory or the clinic." These are the plain objectives of this book.

*J. M. A.*

*January 1967*

# Acknowledgments

I am deeply grateful to several friends for reviewing the manuscript and offering many helpful suggestions. I would like to express my sincere thanks to Drs. Walter C. Alvarez, Robert W. Huntington, Jr., Aims McGuinness, William D. Misbach, Arthur J. Moss, and Stafford L. Warren.

The help and encouragement of Mr. and Mrs. Milton Hart, Mrs. Ethel Miller, Dr. Julia Baker, and Mrs. Emily Gordon have been invaluable.

For several years, my research has been supported by grants of funds from United Cerebral Palsy, Research and Educational Foundation, Multiple Sclerosis Foundation, and National Institutes of Health, United States Public Health Service. I would like to acknowledge my gratitude for this help, which has contributed in large measure to the background of knowledge which is included in this book.

# Acknowledgements

Viruses and Colds
The Modern Plague

# 1 The Complexity of the Common Cold

*Wealth, honour, freedom, beauty, all are his*
*A very king, in short, of kings he is;*
*In wind and limb sound, vigorous, and bold,*
*Except when troubled by a wretched cold.*

—Horace

"Colds" are the most common illnesses of mankind and as such must concern everyone. The Health Interview Survey Program of the United States Public Health Service collects data about acute illnesses and other health topics in a continuing series of weekly household interviews. The results show that there are about 227 million acute coldlike illnesses per year in America. These figures represent individuals who seek medical care or are required to restrict their usual activities for at least one day. Many other minor illnesses or indispositions are not included (see Figure 1).

More important than the actual numbers of acute ill-

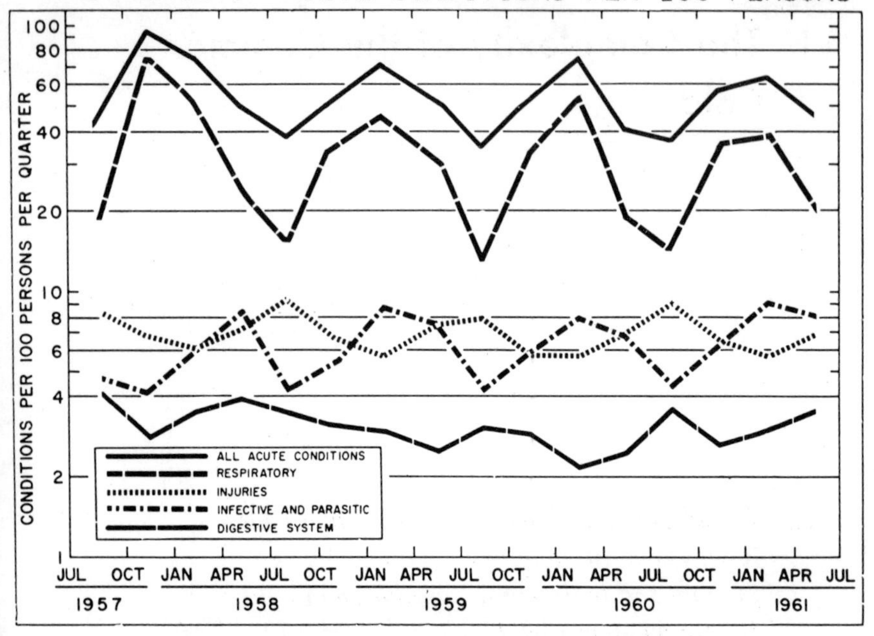


*Figure 1. This graph illustrates the relative importance of respiratory diseases in relation to accidents and other common illnesses such as diarrhea. They account for the great majority of all acute conditions, rising sharply in the winter months. From* Health Statistics, *Series B., No. 33, page 3, Figure 1. U. S. Department of Health, Education, and Welfare, Public Health Service.*

nesses are the consequences of these often-called "nuisance" diseases. These common acute diseases are frequently caused by viruses which may also cause serious illnesses such as pneumonia, heart disease (inflammation of the heart, or carditis), and fever of the brain (encephalitis). "Colds" are really just a mild manifestation of a great many different infecting agents, including the influenza viruses and their cousins known as the parainfluenza viruses, the polioviruses, Coxsackie viruses, ECHO and rhinoviruses, rarely bacteria, and even fungal infections such as "valley fever." When *mild,* they are frequently called "a cold."

Outstanding advances in our ability to find viruses and to grow them have accounted for the greatly increased understanding of the very basic causes of this commonplace illness. The myths surrounding the cause of "colds" are rapidly being dispelled. Apparently, we don't "catch cold" by sitting in a draft, or by living in a cold climate. We acquire the viruses from other human beings who are spraying them in the atmosphere by sneezing, coughing, and talking. Research studies with human volunteers have clearly demonstrated this point. The last word regarding the role of "chilling," however, has not been said. Certain viruses grow more luxuriantly at temperatures a few degrees below normal body temperatures, and it is possible that the chill induces a change in the environment which may trigger the beginning of a "cold." A great deal remains to be learned before we understand the intricacies of this complex problem; many facts, however, are known and should be available to everyone.

The main purpose of this book is to present in as clear a manner as possible the solid and well-established truths concerning our most common health problem. Our ancestors went to bed "as naked as a needil"; but only the hardiest of them survived. The patient is probably the best judge of his state of being. We are all quite familiar with the symptoms and signs of a "cold," as most of us experience one or two a year. Children have many more. Mild symptoms of sneezing and running nose with little or no fever are frequently called "head colds" or "coryza." When the throat, larynx, and bronchial tubes and even the lungs become involved, the term "chest cold" is more common. The physician is often at a loss to make a diagnosis from his findings alone. Volunteers who have been given "colds" are usually the best ones to determine the extent of the illness by their own feelings.

It is obvious that a "cold" is not a simple or clear-cut disease, but a complex of symptoms and signs with many causes, viruses being by far the most common. We must constantly remember that a wide range of symptoms is characteristic of almost all these illnesses. This phenomenon has been referred to as the "clinical spectrum" and may be picturesquely thought of as an "iceberg." That is, much of the actual illness may be inapparent or hidden from view. This fundamental concept is quite essential to keep in mind if we are to acquire a clearer understanding of these diseases.

Emphasis will be placed on some of the serious complications of "colds," or what may be thought of as "aftereffects." These have been referred to in the previous paragraphs as pneumonia, carditis, and encephalitis. Nearly all of the viruses known to effect man may on rare occasions cause inflammation of the brain with serious aftereffects such as convulsions, paralysis, and mental retardation.

Why have we suddenly learned so much about these most common of all illnesses? Advances have come so rapidly that physicians have been overwhelmed by the complexities which little by little are being clarified. Widespread use of the wonder drugs (antibiotics) almost dramatically brought the common bacterial pneumonias and ear infections under control; but unfortunately they have been of little or no avail against primary illnesses usually caused by viruses. These diseases still remain *virtually untouched in incidence and severity.* With the problem of bacterial pneumonia sharply diminished, the viral diseases are more evident, and the term "virus pneumonia" is now popular.

An avalanche of new knowledge followed as a result of our increased ability to study viruses. When it was discovered that these smallest and sometimes lethal enemies could be grown in living cells in test tubes with relative ease, virologists soon discovered more viruses than there were diseases caused by them. Even the virologists were confused. Tissue culture had been known for some time as a delicate method to grow cells, but its adaptation by virologists accounted for the breakthrough that has shaken the biologic sciences by the heels.

The Nobel Prize in medicine was awarded to Dr. John F. Enders and his pediatric associates, Drs. Frederick C. Robbins and Thomas H. Weller, who, working in the Children's Hospital in Boston, demonstrated that viruses could be planted in test tubes that had previously been prepared with growing cells. In a matter of hours or a few days, changes occurred in the tissue cells which were attacked by the viruses. The changes were often characteristic for a particular kind of virus. However when antibodies were added to the culture, these characteristic changes could be prevented, and thus the specific virus might be identified as the cause of the patient's illness.

The ability to grow viruses in glass tubes and bottles in great quantities has made possible the outstanding development of several safe and effective vaccines. The polio vaccines and the vaccines for prevention of measles are the most striking examples. Influenza and adenovirus vaccines are further examples of the rapid progress toward the ultimate goal of prevention.

What can be said about the direct treatment of these common illnesses, particularly those known to be caused by viruses? Although this has been a most discouraging field, fraught with many failures, there is some real hope on the horizon. Probably the most outstanding of these antiviral substances is *interferon,* discovered by two British scientists, Isaacs and Lindenmann, and reported first in 1957. The identification of interferon, which is a substance produced by body cells in response to attack by viruses, was greeted initially with great enthusiasm. It represented another breakthrough in the arduous task of searching for antiviral treatment. This important discovery, however, is still confined to the research laboratory, where the way it works is under intensive study. It is known that it differs from antibodies, which attack germs directly. Interferon in contrast goes into normal cells and protects them from invasion by the virus or prevents viruses from growing in the cell.

A new concept of "recovery" has resulted from this research. It appears that antibodies may have little to do with our getting well from an *initial* viral infection. Interferon and other mechanisms are now considered mainly responsible. The principal role of antibodies is to prevent infection when a germ attacks us for a *second* time. The effectiveness of interferon in preventing disease is striking indeed, but as yet insufficient quantities are available to treat active disease.

Recently a few drugs have been found to have a direct and favorable effect against specific virus diseases. One of these is used in the treatment of infection caused by the herpes virus, which causes fever blisters. Dr. Herbert E. Kaufman demonstrated in 1962 the effectiveness of idoxuridine (IDU) in the treatment of corneal (outer covering of the eye) ulcers due to *herpes simplex* virus. The drug is available and has been used for herpetic infections of the skin such as "cold sores." Recently a new substance to attack viruses has been revealed which is even more potent than IDU. It is called *phagicin,* as it comes from the interaction of *phage* viruses with bacteria. The outlook for direct treatment is much brighter as advances are made in our understanding of the basic workings of viral infections.

■

From this brief introduction it is apparent that what people call "colds" is pretty much their own business, often oversimplified and replete with folklore. Of all the attacking germs that indispose us, viruses are known to play the leading role. Some infect us, and we never know it; others (or the *same* virus) may cause a mild illness, a "common cold," and, unless complicated, recovery is uneventful. It is a fact that in certain individuals, severe symptoms may predominate with signs of laryngitis, bronchitis, or even pneumonia—all caused by the *same* virus. Fortunately many confine their major activity to producing inapparent or mild symptoms. An important new group of viruses responsible for "colds" is known as the *rhinoviruses;* occasionally these may be serious for babies. Nearly all virus illnesses appear to have a spectrum or wide range of symptoms. Different names have been attached over the years—such as "croup," sore throat, virus pneumonia, "the flu," and encephalitis. Patients and human volunteers call these diseases when mild a "headcold" or "chest cold."

Some of the factors which account for the complexity of viral diseases may be explained on the basis of the reaction between the attacking virus and the patient. It is known that age may play a vital and important part in determining the type of illness caused by a virus infection. Certain viruses are more apt to produce a distinct illness in children as opposed to adults. Influenza attacks both children and adults, but in general it can be said that most viruses cause more severe symptoms in infants and young children. Exceptions occur in the instances of chickenpox, measles, and poliomyelitis—which may be much more severe in older individuals than in infancy and early childhood. An illness in infants and young children may be their first experience with the infecting germ. On the other hand, an illness in the adult is often a reinfection and consequently may be milder or even inapparent. Influenza in an Eskimo community was recorded as very severe among the natives who were suffering from this particular illness for the first time. People in the same settlement who had lived for years in more populated centers experienced a mild illness, more than likely related to previous infection.

# 2 The Nature of Acute Respiratory Illnesses and Viruses

The first chapter dealt with the commonness, the complexities, and the seriousness of the common cold. A knowledge of the basic facts will greatly enhance the understanding of these complex illnesses, and it not only will simplify but also should greatly increase the pleasure of learning more about them. Many might still question the over-all significance of colds, and when compared with the pestilences and infections that swept away our ancestors, such as smallpox, the plague, and yellow fever, they do seem insignificant. The importance of these mild illnesses cannot be measured directly, since we are increasingly aware of the fundamental part they play as *initiators* of serious diseases. Colds are usually the first infection, which may begin rather abruptly, sometimes with fever but often without. Illnesses may last from a few hours to a few days; they rarely extend into weeks unless a complication has arisen.

Primary respiratory infections are by far the most common illnesses of man. It has been stated that over 95 per cent of them are caused by viruses, but only in about half of the cases is it possible to make a specific causal diagnosis. Methods for doing this are expensive and time consuming and are rarely pursued except by researchers. Ordinary bacteria that inhabit our nose and throat are the commonest complicators of colds. These germs may infect the sinuses, may occasionally cause infection in the inner ear, or may get into the lung and result in bronchitis and pneumonia. When a baby develops pneumonia or meningitis due to one or more of several common bacteria, it is sometimes easy to forget that the illness started with a cold. A significant quotation from Dr. C. H. Andrewes, Director of the Virus Research Laboratories in England, follows: "Of the legions of bacterial species in man's external and internal environment, only comparatively few ever cause disease." Complications by bacteria can often be detected by the persistence of fever and the development of other symptoms such as headache, earache, increase in cough and in the toxic symptoms of an otherwise mild illness. The glands in the neck may become swollen and tender and indicate the possibility of a bacterial complication. It thus becomes important for the physician, who is called upon daily to diagnose and treat these common diseases, to separate primary symptoms from secondary complications.

Widespread and almost indiscriminate use of drugs, antibiotics in particular, for most of these infections is *not* indicated. When secondary or complicating signs are evident, or even highly suspected, wise choice of an antibiotic can usually be made. The problem is not a simple one to be resolved with a diagnosis of tonsillitis, pharyngitis, or bronchitis, probably due to a virus. It is important to try to determine the cause and make as accurate a diagnosis as possible, based on a good history, a physical examination, and certain laboratory tests when needed.

A knowledge of the various possibilities, the season, and the epidemic nature of many of these diseases is extremely important in arriving at a diagnosis. Just as with measles, chickenpox, and mumps, all due to specific viruses, it is necessary to evaluate the common features of many of the newer virus diseases and make a practical working diagnosis. Much of the contents of this book will be devoted to the common signs and symptoms of these diseases in order to gain a clearer understanding of causes, the full spectrum of illness, and serious complications.

An example of what we're talking about is influenza. A diagnosis of "the flu" is often made, not only by the patient but by the doctor, particularly when associated with the symptoms of generalized aching and weakness. Influenza is an epidemic virus disease, usually occurring in the winter months. It is distinguished by a sudden onset of fever, sore throat, and weakness. Running nose and cough are frequently present. A diagnosis of influenza or "the flu" is made and reported every day in various communities of our wide land; however, influenza is known to occur in epidemics which begin sharply and end sharply, lasting but a few weeks. For all practical purposes the diagnosis should be confined to epidemic periods; and although many viral infections simulate influenza, the diagnosis should rarely if ever be made. During an epidemic most acute illnesses are due to the influenza virus, but outside of an epidemic period there is less than one chance in a hundred that an acute coldlike illness is truly influenza.

The problem isn't one of discovering the viruses causing illness, but of defining their role in producing disease. It is possible to obtain three or four different viruses from the same child on the same day. Viruses may invade us and cause an illness which is totally inapparent. At the time of influenza epidemics many people may be infected, as shown by blood tests, and yet experience no illness.

This important concept may be further illustrated by both poliomyelitis and tuberculosis. It is known that most older children and adults have polio two or three times and probably not one in a hundred is aware of the illness, or associates it with a serious disease like poliomyelitis. Persons who develop a positive tuberculin test are usually totally unaware of when this happened. A certain percentage, however, suffer from a "head cold" or a "chest cold" which may last for several weeks. It may have been at this time that they were infected by the tubercle bacillus and several weeks later developed a positive tuberculin test. There is good evidence that most positive tests are acquired without any knowledge of serious illness on the part of the individual.

It is clear that viruses play the dominant role as causes of common respiratory disease. What are the viruses? How do they multiply and survive from one person to another? Primarily as a result of our increased ability to study and work with viruses, a new science known as "molecular biology" is evolving. One of the most intriguing mysteries of nature is not only the way chemical compounds make up the living creature, but the ability of this living organism to reproduce itself. The chemical that governs heredity is a substance known as deoxyribonucleic acid or DNA. DNA is important to everyone, as it is actually the basic material for the transfer of biologic information from parent to child. In 1962 the Nobel Prize in medicine was awarded to Dr. James Watson of Harvard University, to Dr. Maurice Wilkins of Kings College, London, and to Dr. Francis Crick of Cambridge University, whose studies have revealed the very structure and function of DNA.

There are two kinds of nucleic acid found in the cells of our body; also in germs and viruses. One is DNA, mentioned above, and the other is RNA (ribonucleic acid). They are similar in many respects, as the molecule of both consists of long chains of chemicals known as nucleotides. These are linked together by sugar and a chemical known as phosphate. The RNA molecules consist of a single strand, whereas the DNA molecules are nearly always double stranded but rarely may occur in a single strand. This might be pictured as a ladder in which these chains of alternating sugar and phosphate form the sides which are tied together by rungs. The ladder is then twisted in a spiral to form what is known as a double helix (Figure 2). It is known that the DNA molecule stores genetic information and controls the manufacture of protein substances on which the whole life process and growth depends. Vi-

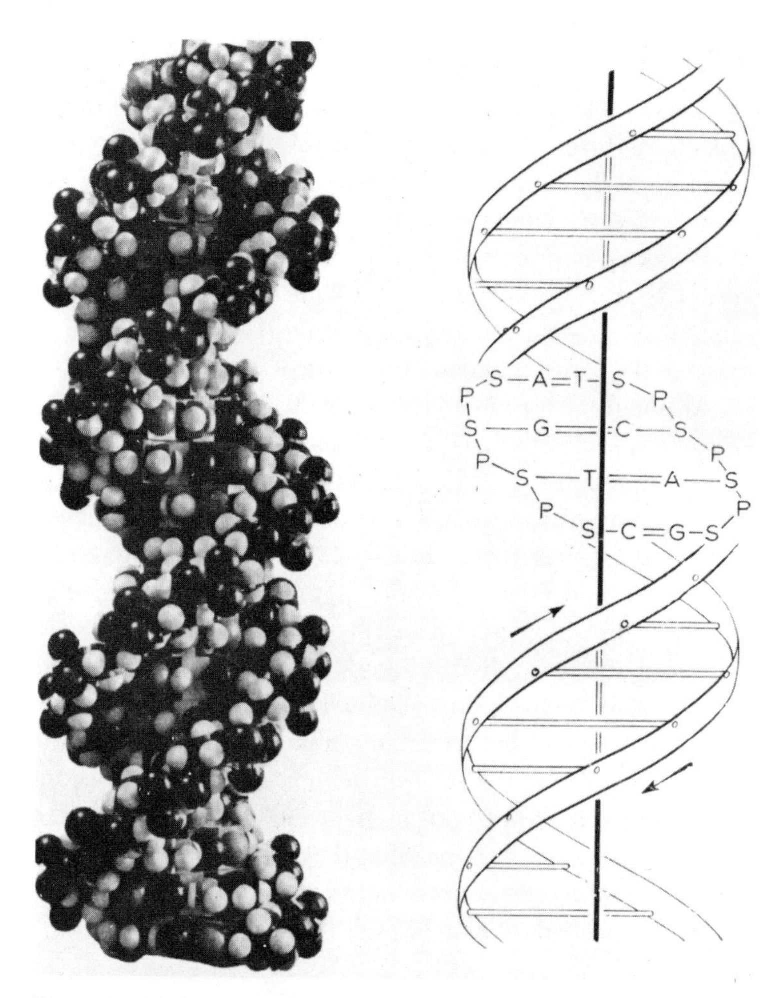


*Figure 2. A diagrammatic representation of the DNA molecule as proposed by Watson and Crick. This twisted structure is called a double helix. By permission of Academic Press Inc.,* The Viruses, *edited by Burnet and Stanley.*

ruses are made up of these nucleic acids and possess one or the other type of nucleic acid, never both.

These most important chemicals of life have two main jobs to perform. The first is to control the process of reproducing itself in order that genetic information may be transferred to daughter cells. The second responsibility is to pass this information over to the factories in the cell in order that the proper materials will be manufactured. In the latter process the RNA molecules themselves participate in the transfer and manufacture of protein.

Although viruses are known chiefly because they cause disease in man, animals, and plants, research and study of this simplest form of life has contributed to a better understanding of the very "secret of life" itself. The nucleic acids, DNA and RNA, which make up the structure of every cell and thus the whole organism, are contained in the nuclei of the egg and sperm when they unite to begin the formation of a living thing. Understanding this basic mechanism, by means of which all life is evolved on earth, can lead to great dividends for mankind. Scientists may be able to determine the basis of *thought* itself. Memory consists of information stored in giant molecules according to the genetic code. It is possible that we may learn to control inheritance and hence the destiny of plants and animals and perhaps of man himself.

■

With over two hundred viruses capable of causing acute illnesses in man, it becomes important to try to arrange these in some logical manner if we are to identify diseases according to their *causes* rather than by the anatomical areas of the body which may be involved. Virologists have grouped viruses in an attempt to work out a classification that would be helpful in naming certain diseases. Viruses are grouped according to their chemical and physical properties based on the core material, whether it is DNA or RNA. Their size also is useful in placing them in certain groups. There are four DNA groups and four RNA groups, but a few viruses remain outside awaiting further identification. The finding of many new viruses does not prove that they cause disease. For some time, the wide range of symptoms caused by one virus has been recognized. It may overwhelm one person, as with bulbar polio, or it may infect another person without any sign of illness. Also, a disease such as virus pneumonia may be produced by many different viruses. A further example of the spectrum might be found in infections caused by the Coxsackie B viruses. They may produce mild, coldlike illnesses or high fever with pain in the chest, known as pleurodynia or "devil's grippe." The same virus may cause meningitis, and in babies the inflammation of the brain and heart may be fatal (See Chapter IX).

These groups or families are very large, ranging from as many as ten to a hundred different viruses in certain categories. Although confusing, it will be helpful in the long run to think about diseases in terms of *causes*, rather than whether they involve the nose, throat, tonsils, or bronchial tubes. Terms such as tonsillitis, nasal pharyngitis, and bronchitis become meaningless when one is considering the proper treatment and eventual outlook for the patient. It is important to know if we are dealing with influenza, adenovirus, or a streptococcal infection of the throat or a combination of agents. It is true that the same symptoms may be caused by many different germs. The doctor is therefore frequently hard put to make a specific *causal* diagnosis. On the other hand, by knowing the characteristics of many of these illnesses, whether they occur in epidemics and at what season of the year, plus the aid of certain laboratory tests, it is possible to arrive at a practical working diagnosis. We can no longer be content to label a disease as simply tonsillitis or laryngitis. Great progress is being made in the rapid diagnosis of some of these common diseases, many of which overlap and simulate each other.

On the accompanying reference table a general grouping of these illnesses gives some idea of the total number of the known viruses, most of which may cause varying degrees of acute respiratory disease. The first group is called *Myxovirus* and includes influenza and the parainfluenza viruses; the measles virus and respiratory syncytial (RS) virus also are included in this large family.

The second group, known as *Adenovirus* also produces adenoiditis and tonsillitis and causes conjunctivitis as well.

The third large group has been designated as *Picornavirus*. This group includes the polioviruses, Coxsackie and ECHO viruses as well as the new rhinoviruses. The latter agents probably account for a considerable proportion of colds, particularly in adults. It must be emphasized again that nearly *all* of these virus diseases *when mild* may simulate an illness which people call "colds."

## Acute Respiratory Diseases of Man*

| GROUP | VIRUSES | DISEASES |
|---|---|---|
| *Myxovirus* (*RNA*) | Influenza (A, B, C) | Influenza, croup, "colds," and virus pneumonia |
| | Parainfluenza (1–4) | Acute respiratory disease with fever, croup, "colds," and virus pneumonia |
| | Measles | Acute respiratory diseases with rash, rarely pneumonia and encephalitis |
| | Respiratory Syncytial | Acute respiratory disease, "colds" in adults; bronchiolitis and pneumonia in infants |
| *Adenovirus* (*DNA*) | Adenoviruses (1–31) | Acute respiratory disease with fever<br>"Common colds"<br>Virus pneumonia<br>Cancer in hamsters |
| *Picornavirus* (*RNA*) | Poliovirus (1–3) | Poliomyelitis<br>Acute respiratory disease with fever<br>"Summer colds" |
| | Coxsackie A (1–23) | Pharyngitis with vesicles<br>Meningitis and "colds" |
| | Coxsackie B (1–6) | Chest pain and inflammation of the heart<br>Meningitis and "colds" |
| | ECHO virus (1–32) | Meningitis and "colds"<br>Diarrhea (newborn) |
| | Rhinovirus (83 or more) | "Common colds" (rhinitis, coryza in adults)<br>More serious respiratory illness in children such as bronchitis and pneumonia |
| *Mycoplasma* | *M. pneumoniae* (bacterium) | Acute respiratory disease, bronchitis, and pneumonia |

* *Other viruses causing respiratory diseases in man are reoviruses and lymphocytic choriomeningitis virus.*

# 3 The Lungs and How They Work; Tonsils and Adenoids

Thomas Willis (1622–75) studied the structure of the lung by injecting colored liquids. He gave one of the earliest descriptions of the pulmonary tree, which he clearly illustrated in Figure 3. Although recognized as the outstanding practicing physician of his time, he is best known today for his contributions to anatomy and experimental medicine. Willis described the arteries which circle the base of the brain; they still go by his name. A passage from his elegy describes the genius of the man:

*Thou knewst the wonderous art*
*And order of each part*
*In the whole lump, how every sense*
*Contributes to the health's defense.*

Acute, coldlike illnesses affect the breathing passages, which make up one of the most vital systems of our body.

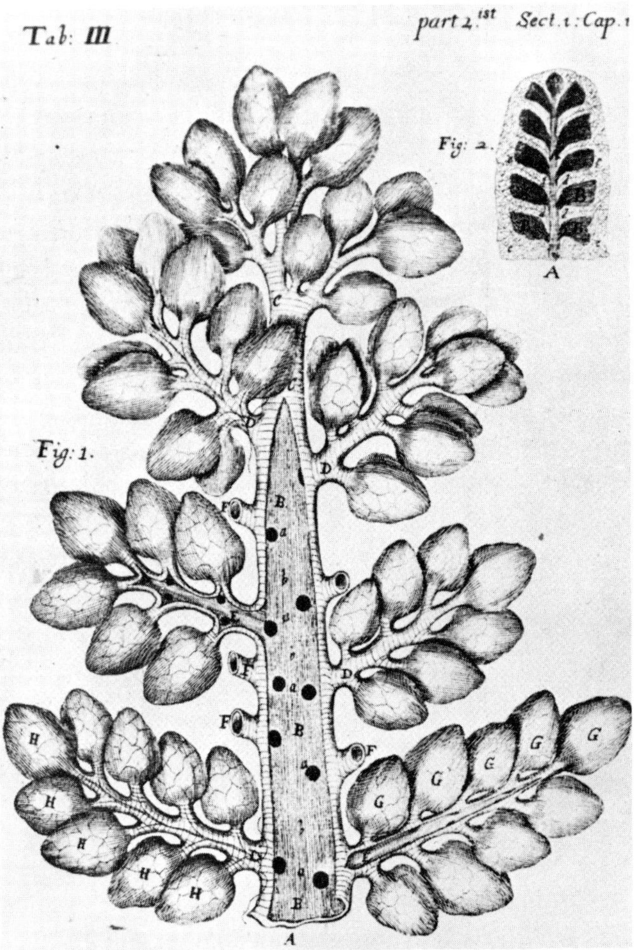

*Figure 3. A lobe of the lung showing its subdivisions. The main stem is a bronchus, which sends off smaller branches, or bronchioles. These divide to form "little bladders" or air sacs called alveoli, labeled H and G.*

They may be affected mildly as with a "running" nose or critically as with pneumonia. Every minute of our lives, from the first breath, we are dependent upon the heart to pump blood through the lungs to get essential oxygen. The breathing passages are like a tree and literally may be compared in all their various parts. It is known to doctors as "the pulmonary tree," the roots of which are comparable to the sinuses and the tubes leading to the inner ears. The base of the tree is the throat. The trunk is the windpipe (trachea) which divides into two main branches, called bronchi. These in turn divide many times into smaller and smaller branches called bronchioles. From these the millions of little air sacs or leaves come off. The leaves are called alveoli. When they become inflamed, the condition is called pneumonia. The lung of the adult human being contains approximately 300 million little air sacs.

Figure 4 is a picture of part of a single air sac or leaf, taken with an electron miscroscope. It shows a dumbbell-shaped red blood cell and where it has to go to get its oxygen. The membranes that form the edge of the breathing sac have been clearly shown for the first time by the electron microscope. The red blood cell, loaded with oxygen, goes back to the left side of the heart to be pumped out to the brain and other organs. It is not difficult to understand how vital it is that this complicated machinery be kept in good working order.

Why do we cough? Irritating substances such as dust will produce a cough; but the most common cause is our own secretions which accumulate in the air passages, nose, throat, and bronchial tubes. This occurs when infection causes inflammation of the surfaces. The little trap door

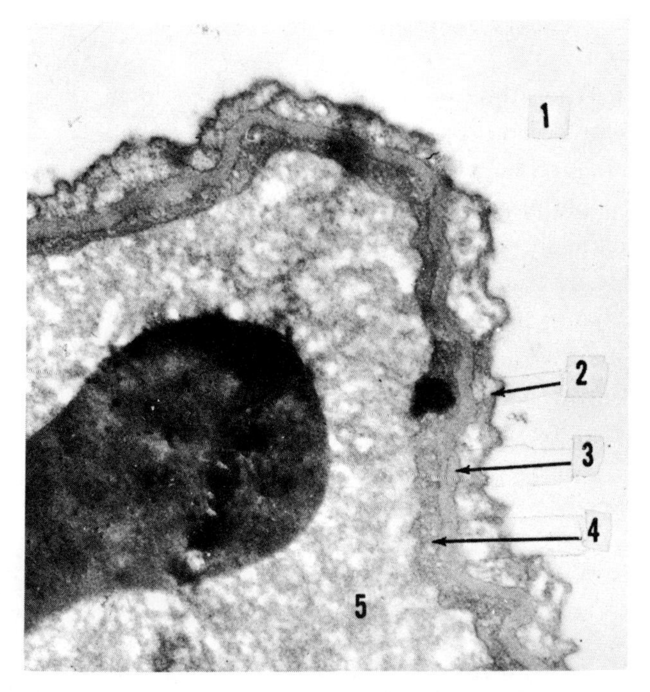


*Figure 4. Electron microscopic photograph of the wall of the air sac or alveolus, showing the various layers (2–4) between the air space (1) and a small blood vessel (5) which contains a red blood cell (large dark area). Magnified 30,000 times. By permission of The Macmillan Company,* Newer Virus Diseases, *copyright © 1960 by John M. Adams. (Courtesy of Drs. Clayton Loosli and Richard F. Baker, University of Southern California School of Medicine).*

(epiglottis) at the top of the windpipe closes and a forceful expiration results in a cough.

The secretions that result from colds accumulate in the nose and throat and may be inhaled into the lower air passages, causing bronchitis and pneumonia. Nearly all pneumonia is caused by inhaling or choking on infected secretions from the nose and throat.

When the individual is placed face down, the secretions tend to run out instead of into the lungs. Cough is often relieved by placing the patient in this position, and pneumonia may actually be prevented. A side-view X ray of a baby shows the downward slope of the main air passage when the child is placed in the prone position. It is frequently referred to as "postural drainage." It is, in addition, the most *natural* position for sleep, and, with a firm mattress below the baby, it is the *safest* position for sleep (See figure 8A, p. 96).

*The Boke of Chyldren* by Thomas Phaire was the first book in pediatrics ever written by an Englishman. It was

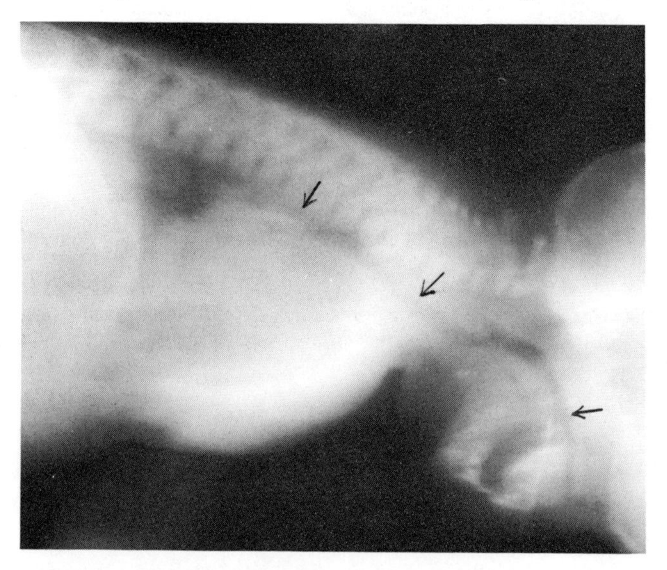

*Figure 5. An X ray of a baby taken from the side to show the windpipe and its downward slope when the baby is placed in the prone or face-down position. By permission of The Macmillan Company,* Newer Virus Diseases, *copyright © 1960 by John M. Adams.*

published in 1545. Undoubtedly he was the first to write about the importance of posture in the treatment of cough. A passage entitled "Of the Cough" follows:

> The cough in childre for the moste part, procedeth either of a cold, or by reason of reumes, descending from the head into the pipes of the longes or the breast, and that is moste comonly by ouermuche aboudauce of milke corrupting the stomack and brayne: therfore in that case, it is good to fede the childe with a more slender diete, & to annointe the head ouer with hony, and nowe and than to presse his tong with your fynger, holdyng downe hys head that the reumes may issue, for by that meanes the cause of the cough shall runne out of his mouthe, and auoyde the childe of many noughty and slimy humours whiche done, many times the paciente amendeth without any further helpe of medicine.

Sir William Osler said, "Sore throat in children may be the only evidence of acute articular rheumatism or infantile paralysis. They enter through the tonsils." *

The tonsils are situated in the throat in small pockets on either side of the tongue in the very rear of the mouth. Their actual purpose in life was not very clear until recent discoveries in the field of immunology revealed the very important role they play in keeping us well.

The tonsils stand at the gateway of attack by viruses, bacteria, and other microbes. We lead a life of "coexistence" with the myriad of microorganisms in our environment. The tonsils and adenoids, which form a ring of defense in the nose and throat, are waging the battle every

*Bean, William Bennett, ed., *Sir William Osler: Aphorisms from his Bedside Teachings and Writings.* (New York: Henry Schuman, Inc.).

day. When we get sick with a sore throat and fever, the invasion is usually due to a new germ (that is, new to the individual), such as the Asian influenza virus which appeared out of the blue in 1957. Millions were attacked, and the virus spread around the world causing a pandemic of influenza. Although many people died during the epidemic (78,000 in the United States), most recovered owing to the heroic battle waged by the various defenses of the body.

Tonsils and adenoids are made up almost entirely of the lymphocytes and plasma cells, which are known to manufacture antibodies. They are, however, only a part of a very elaborate network of cells and tissues concerned with keeping us well. The thymus gland, until recently considered quite useless, plays a vital role in mobilizing the fighting cells which go to the spleen, tonsils, and even the appendix. The plasma cells that make the antibodies are found in vertebrates and not in lower forms of life. A very basic mechanism, however, does exist even in plants, and this is the ability of all cells to make a substance called "interferon" (discussed in Chapter I). It works inside the cells, where antibiotics are not very effective. The virus or germ is coated with a protective protein material, which prevents multiplication or reproduction of new virus and so the infection stops.

The tonsils and adenoids are intimately concerned with nearly every disease discussed in this book. They are the first line of defense, forming a buffer which keeps the infection under control, and thus only mild or inapparent illness results—often referred to as a cold, a sore throat, or a touch of the flu. When the infection is virulent, the defenses may be overwhelmed and complications become evident. For some reason, our bodies manufacture less interferon when attacked by virulent germs. This may be why they are so virulent.

The commonest complications of acute infections in the nose and throat are due to invasion of the glands in the neck, sinuses, and inner ears. These may be the result of the initial virus infection or due to bacteria which are lurking around waiting for the opportunity to attack. They may even work together and spread beyond the sinuses and ears, resulting in mastoiditis or meningitis. Bronchitis and pneumonia are also important complications.

The indications for removing "life-saving organs" like tonsils and adenoids must be clearly defined and serious thought given to the decision. Ordinarily the operation is not considered to be a dangerous one, but a few hundred children (200 to 300) die every year in this country in direct association with tonsillectomy. Deaths are usually due to anesthesia or to hemorrhage. Rarely a lung abscess may follow the operation if infected material is aspirated into the lung.

There are only a few clear indications for the operation, which usually includes the adenoids as well as the tonsils. Serious obstruction may be caused by the adenoids, which may block breathing through the nose and obstruct drainage from the inner ear. An abscess may occur around the tonsils, sometimes called quinsy. When this occurs, which it does very rarely these days, an operation may be necessary if adequate attempts to clear the infection with simple drainage and antibiotics have failed. Chronic tonsillitis or frequent recurring attacks may be an indication for surgery, but only after a thorough study and a trial of adequate antibacterial drugs.

There are many types of streptococci. Following an infection by a particular type, immunity results, so that it is possible that a new infection is responsible for what may seem like a recurrence of the previous illness (see Chapter XIII for more detailed discussion of "strep" infections.)

Tuberculosis of the glands in the neck may rarely be a reason to consider tonsillectomy. Here again an adequate trial of antituberculosis drugs should be made before surgery is considered.

A final statement regarding conditions for which tonsillectomy is often employed without benefit needs more emphasis. Recurring common colds and running nose, often accompanied by a poor appetite and failure to gain weight, are *not* an indication for surgery. As the child gets older, these problems frequently clear up. Sometimes the tonsils become very large, but do not cause symptoms. This apparent reason for removal is rarely sufficient to warrant such a procedure and may even be a favorable sign of a strong defense by the body. Many times the tonsils will appear tremendous and actually touch each other if the child is suffering from an acute infection. When seen weeks later, however, they will often be reduced to an unimpressive size and enthusiasm for removal will have subsided.

When an operation has been decided on, certain steps

should be taken to make sure the risks are negligible and the probability of benefit is assured. A blood abnormality should be ruled out, but if one is present, proper steps should be taken to avoid excess bleeding. For example, a white blood count showed glandular fever or infectious mononucleosis (Chapter XI) in a child about to have a tonsillectomy, and the operation was postponed. The postponing of surgery often results in favorable changes which make an operation unnecessary.

The operation of adenotonsillectomy varies widely from one community to another and in different economic groups. At Eton School in England, about 80 per cent of the boys have had their tonsils removed. In the city of Sheffield, the incidence is less than one half of one per cent. The same striking differences can be found in the United States of America. The conclusions of recent studies "although showing beyond doubt that by and large adenotonsillectomy has no favorable influence on the health of children, cannot be interpreted as proving that the operation does not help in certain isolated cases. The physician will do well to recommend against operation except in very special instances." *

* Bakwin (see Selected References, p. 160)

# 4 Epidemic Influenza and Its Prevention

> . . . it began with a roughness of the jaws, small cough, then a strong fever, with a pain of the head, back and legs; some felt as though they were over the breast and had a weight on the stomach; all which continued to the third day at the farthest; there the fever went off with a sweat or bleeding at the nose. In some few, it turned to pleurisy, or fatal peri pneumony. . . .

This clear description of influenza in 1557 was recorded by Thomas Short and is wholly applicable to influenza as we know it today. The earliest date on record for pandemic influenza is 1173; since then, several pandemics of influenza have occurred at irregular intervals. The most outstanding was the pandemic of 1918–19, which was responsible for 20 million deaths. "Pandemic" refers to a worldwide epidemic and does not mean severity of illness. The most recent pandemic occurred in the fall of 1957 and the early months of 1958. It is commonly referred to as Asian or A2 influenza.

It was not until 1933 that influenza was proved beyond doubt to be caused by a virus. Prior to that time it was identified largely on the basis of the clinical features and its striking tendency to occur in epidemics. Influenza has been known for centuries in Europe, America, and Asia as a disease that spreads rapidly through populations of the entire country at periodic intervals. Reasons for the spread of influenza throughout the world are not clearly known today. The contagiousness of influenza was recognized by Robert Johnson, who described the details of the influenza epidemic of 1789 and called attention to the speed with which it spread from one community to another. He expressed difficulty in accounting for the rapid advance of this disease at a time when travel was very limited and stated that "the disease often does arise from some vicious quality of the air or exhalation in it, as well as from a matter arising from the body of a man labouring under disease."

The many hair-raising and tragic stories surrounding epidemic influenza must still give us pause for thought. We have no assurance today that influenza can be controlled, and epidemics are still occurring at regular intervals. The pandemic of 1918 was the most severe experience with this disease history has recorded. It began in early spring in Spain, where it appeared suddenly and after a brief course subsided without leaving a trace. Similar epidemics appeared in England, France, and the United States in April of 1918; and, at the same time,

Japan and China recorded a three-day fever similar to influenza. The first wave was mild compared with the second wave, which occurred in the fall of 1918.

Influenza appeared in many parts of the world at the same time and by October was world-wide in its distribution. Although in general considered mild, two serious forms made their appearance. The first was an illness characterized by a sudden onset, with acute inflammation of the lungs, accompanied by blueness and death in a few hours or days. The second type developed on the fourth or fifth day of what appeared to be a slight illness or a cold, at which time pneumonia became evident and resulted in death or a long convalescence.

As has been pointed out, epidemics are due to influenza viruses, types A and B. Type A epidemics occur approximately every two or three years; epidemics caused by influenza type B tend to occur at longer intervals, usually four to six years.

Because influenza is diagnosed daily when there is no known epidemic, it becomes important to consider it seriously in any discussion of common coldlike illnesses. In nonepidemic periods acute diseases which are due to many other viruses are frequently referred to as "the flu"; and all of these in their milder forms have been called a cold. During an influenza epidemic as many as 25 to 50 per cent of persons are infected, as shown by increasing antibodies in their blood. However, *actual* illnesses in the same community may be no more than 5 to 10 per cent. A moment of calculation quickly indicates that in a city of a million people, 50,000 to 100,000 may experience an acute illness, whereas 400,000 to 500,000 may actually be infected by the virus. The over-all death rate during influenza epidemics often rises tenfold in a community for the limited period of the epidemic.

The discovery of the influenza virus in 1933 marked a very important point in understanding this world-wide scourge. A tremendous amount of research followed the great pandemic of 1918–19, and, although the virus cause of the disease was strongly suspected at that time, proof was lacking. Many experiments were carried out to establish the contagiousness of influenza, but for the most part they failed to do so. In the light of our present knowledge it is difficult to understand the failure of these transmission experiments, except for the fact that the volunteers may have had a previous mild or inapparent illness which protected them.

The influenza bacillus of Pfeiffer was considered for many years to be the cause of influenza. The studies of Dr. Richard E. Shope in 1931 of swine influenza provided a clear demonstration of the role of bacteria in this disease. A germ very similar to the influenza bacillus was found in swine, and it could be found consistently in sick animals; however, when this germ was given to other susceptible animals no illness occurred. Thus it was discovered that the bacillus was not the sole cause of swine influenza and that a virus was responsible for the initial mild illness. When combined, the two agents *acting together* produced a most serious and frequently fatal form of swine influenza.

Although the cause of the 1918–19 pandemic of influenza will probably never be proved, it is possible that swine influenza, which was prevalent that year, was in some way related to the pandemic in human beings. Survivors from that epidemic have antibodies in their blood against swine influenza. The swine virus is similar to type A in human beings, which is recognized as the most important and most common cause of this disease.

The recent Asian influenza epidemic has some unusual and interesting features. It had its origin late in February of 1957 in southwest China, spreading from there to Yunnan province; it was reported throughout much of the Orient during the spring months. It appeared first in the United States in the middle of May among military personnel arriving at San Diego, California, from the Pacific area. Following its introduction in May into America, small outbreaks occurred at summer camps and conventions. In this manner the seeding process took place throughout the United States prior to the development of the widespread epidemic in October 1957.

The virus was readily identified as type A prior to the start of the epidemic. It appeared to be quite different in its characteristics from the usual type A. This suggested that the amount of immunity or protection in the world was probably at a low level and that a pandemic might develop. The disease reached pandemic proportions in the fall and early winter months, then subsided, only to be followed by a second wave in January, February, and March of 1958. The world experience was relatively mild, with illnesses that averaged approximately three days with few complications.

Public Health Service figures gathered from 108 cities are shown in Figure 6. It clearly demonstrates the two phases of the epidemic and the sharp increase in deaths throughout the United States. Although the epidemic was considered mild, the Surgeon General's statistics estimated that between 30 and 50 million Americans suffered from the Asian variety of influenza and that more than 78,000 deaths could be directly attributed to the disease.

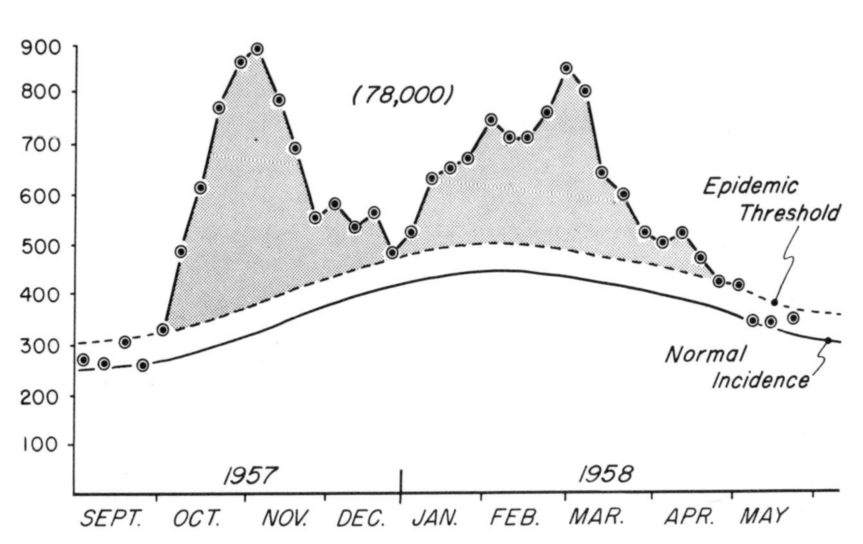


*Figure 6. A graph showing the increased mortality (from 300 deaths per week to 900 per week) in 108 cities in the United States during the Asian influenza epidemic of 1957–58. It illustrates the epidemic nature of influenza. From the United States Public Health Service. By permission of The Macmillan Company,* Newer Virus Diseases, *copyright © 1960 by John M. Adams.*

A heroic effort was made on the part of the government with the cooperation of pharmaceutical manufacturing concerns to prepare a vaccine against Asian influenza. Twelve million doses became available prior to the main epidemic, and there is evidence that the vaccine played a significant role in controlling the severity of this pandemic. Antibiotics undoubtedly helped to control or prevent many of the serious bacterial complications which so commonly accompany influenza.

The striking experience of Dr. Richard Herrmann and associates illustrates clearly that although influenza has been considered a mild and unimportant disease, it may be serious and cause sudden death. These doctors reported 23 sudden deaths occurring in the vicinity of Denver, Colorado, during the height of the Asian influenza epidemic from October 3 to 20, 1957. Four infants, all less than 3 months of age, died suddenly in that short 17-day period. This represents a very high mortality in this infant age group, as no more than five or six patients were involved in any other ten-year age period to account for the 23 deaths.

Another rare but striking feature of Asian flu was encephalitis or "brain fever," which appeared in close association with the epidemic. The symptoms in the classic form of influenza are remarkably uniform. The onset of the disease is usually sudden and characterized by high fever, particularly in infants, where it may range to 104 or 105 degrees Fahrenheit on the first day of illness. Marked lassitude is a striking feature and almost uniformly patients complain of sore throat. The symptoms recorded by Short in 1557 (see the beginning of this chapter) are still the predominant ones in recent epidemics.

The Fourth National Boy Scout Jamboree held at Valley Forge in July 1957 produced one of the early epidemics of the Asian type of influenza. Fever, headache, cough, and sore throat were the most common complaints among the boys. A fairly high percentage also complained of general discomfort and prostration. Muscle aches and pain in the stomach were important features. Red throats were recorded in three quarters of the boys. Inflammation of the eyes and running nose were frequent symptoms. As many as one fifth had signs of inflammation in the chest, which in several instances was confirmed by X ray as a spot of pneumonia.

Dr. Clayton Loosli and associates recorded the clinical characteristics of Asian influenza among naval recruits and emphasized the abrupt high fever with chilliness, malaise, headache, muscle aches, cough, and scratchy throat as the most significant symptoms. They were successful in finding the Asian influenza virus in the majority of their patients, and 80 per cent showed evidence of infection by blood tests.

At the present time vaccination appears to be the most hopeful method for the control of human influenza. The search for effective drugs against the influenza virus has up to now failed to show promise of controlling influenza epidemics. Recently, however, an antiviral drug known as *amantadine* may prove useful in prevention but not in treatment of the Asian type of influenza. In one study involving nearly eight hundred healthy volunteers, the incidence of disease among the group treated with amantadine was 1 per cent, as compared with 4 per cent among the group failing to receive the drug. The mechanism of action apparently is one that prevents the virus from entering the cells of the body, and no evidence of toxic effects has been seen.

Killed vaccine given under the skin is the main method of prevention employed in the United States today. Vaccines in the past have varied greatly in their effectiveness due largely to the changing character of the influenza virus. There are several strains of influenza A and a few of B that are employed in the preparation of vaccine, and when they are used against the same strain of virus, good protection is the result. Vaccination programs in civilian and military populations have been shown to be effective in protecting 60 to 80 per cent of those vaccinated. However, despite these results, there has never been wide civilian acceptance. Changing types and strains have altered the effectiveness of the vaccines, and reactions are sometimes unpleasant.

There are two different approaches to the problem of immunization against influenza. The first is based on the inactivated or killed virus, which is injected below the skin, and the second consists of spraying weakened living viruses into the nose. Russian investigators have reported success with the inhalation of influenza antiserum prepared in horses. There is a high risk of sensitizing the individual to horse serum. They have also employed live virus given by nose. The disadvantage of these methods is the risk of producing severe illness in children and the chance that using many different viruses may result in the interference of one live virus with another.

Outbreaks of influenza A2, which is now the name for Asian influenza, occurred in 1962–63 in many areas of the United States with the exception of the West Coast. The following year influenza A2 was widely prevalent on the West Coast, and because of these two consecutive years in which influenza A caused epidemics in the United States, it could be predicted ahead of time that a major outbreak would not be experienced in the winter months of 1964–65. Influenza B produced a few epidemics in the United States in 1961–62, and Japan experienced an epidemic during 1963–64. On the basis of the cyclic nature of influenza A, the epidemic of A2 early in 1966 was successfully forecasted. It would appear unlikely, however, in the view of the Public Health Service Advisory Committee, that major epidemics of Influenza B will occur in the near future; limited outbreaks may be expected. Recently discovered strains are now put into the vaccine, which has also been concentrated and thus offers promise of more effective protection.

Immunization is recommended for certain individuals who may be expected to have the highest mortality from epidemic influenza. These include people of all ages who suffer from chronic diseases such as those that involve the heart and kidneys. Likewise patients with chronic lung disease, such as asthma and bronchitis or tuberculosis, should be protected. Older age groups (in which deaths have been the highest in past epidemics) as well as pregnant women (who also experience an increased risk from influenza) should receive the vaccine.

For these special groups it is recommended that vaccination be carried out as soon as possible after September 1, to be completed by mid-December. It takes about two weeks to develop immunity after being vaccinated; therefore, it is important that immunization be carried out if possible before influenza occurs in a particular community. Those who have not been vaccinated recently should receive a shot under the skin, and this should be followed by a second dose in approximately two months. Even a single dose will afford some protection and may be followed by a booster injection as early as two weeks in order to increase its effectiveness.

For adults and children over 12 years of age the regular dose is recommended. It is cut in half for children between 6 and 12 years and reduced even further for children from 3 months to 5 years. The dose may also be divided and given one or two weeks apart, to be followed by a third injection in two months. Vaccines are prepared from viruses which are grown in eggs and therefore should not be administered to those who are sensitive to eggs or egg products. A new vaccine eliminates many of the flulike symptoms of previous vaccines and is much more protective even in small doses. It is unique because it contains only the active protein material of the virus. It has been called "split virus" influenza vaccine. Follow your doctor's recommendation.

■

To summarize, influenza is an acute respiratory disease caused by three different types of viruses. The incubation period is short, from one to two days, and illness is characterized by a sudden onset of fever, sore throat, and general aches and pains. The disease lasts about two to four days unless complicated by other germs. It is difficult to distinguish any single case of influenza from other acute illnesses, particularly in the early stages, but when groups of cases occur it can be recognized by the distinct features of influenza and by its tendency to occur in epidemics. Prevention of influenza is well established by means of killed virus vaccines, and protection ranges from 60 to 80 per cent. Treatment consists largely of rest and attention to symptoms as well as a careful watch for complications. When they arise, a wise choice of antibiotics should be made and administered.

# 5 Croup and RS Viruses

The parainfluenza viruses, of which there are four different types, are the first cousins of influenza. They belong in the same large family and are responsible in part at least for "croupy" illnesses, particularly in infants. When sprayed into the throat of human volunteers, they cause a mild illness similar to the common cold. The human volunteer story is interesting—almost exciting—because it represents one of the earliest successful attempts with a known virus to transmit colds to human beings. It also shows that *age* may be important in the seriousness of illness. Infants may have laryngitis and even pneumonia, whereas adults, many of whom have antibodies, get an illness which everyone agrees is a common cold.

In 1958 researchers at the National Institutes of Health reported their results on a trial infection in human volunteers. Thirty-two healthy men, ranging in age from 21 to

46, were given type 2 parainfluenza virus that had been obtained from a baby with acute laryngitis. The serum of all of the men was studied before the experiment started, and most of them showed evidence of type 2 antibodies and therefore were presumed to have had a previous illness caused by this particular virus.

The volunteers were separated and examined daily by two physicians. After five days, when none of the men became ill, the researchers gave up, and the men were released from isolation. The next day, however, six of them reported an acute illness. Immediately all of the volunteers were again segregated, and several others became ill. All of these illnesses were mild; the men recovered uneventfully in two to three days. The symptoms were described as coldlike, with some obstruction of the nose and nasal discharge. Coughing and sneezing were prominent symptoms. A few complained of sore throat, headache, and eye discomfort or chest pain. Hoarseness was present in occasional men. When examined, their throats were red with swelling, particularly on the first day of symptoms. Other common findings were runny nose with inflamed tonsils. Some reported increased tearing and mild inflammation of the eyes; "hay fever" was recorded in four individuals. Over half of the volunteers developed a clear-cut illness, and these same viruses were found in their throats. The virus which was inoculated was also found in about half of the men who did not get sick, so there seemed to be little doubt that their *inapparent* illness was caused by the *same* germ.

The story does not end here! When the men were released from isolation on the fifth day just prior to the onset of their symptoms, during that short break of one day, others in the institution were exposed to them. Eight days following this event, an outbreak of a coldlike illness occurred in the general population of the institution; 18 individuals not included in the study became ill with a mild illness, typical of that produced in the volunteers. The *same* virus was again found. The researchers were able to conclude that the parainfluenza virus may cause mild respiratory disease in adults as well as a more severe acute illness in small children. Although the illness was mild, they considered the mildness was related to the fact that many of the volunteers had evidence of a previous experience with this virus. It is clear that this agent must occupy a prominent place among the causes of the "common cold" in both adults and children.

Sendai virus first recovered from mice in Japan has been classified as parainfluenza, type 1. It is considered by the Japanese to be the cause of pneumonia in newborn babies and also will produce pneumonia in pigs. The virus has rarely been recovered in other countries, although antibodies have been shown to be present in the blood serum of human beings from many places in the world.

Type 2 virus, just discussed in the volunteer study, frequently causes a crouplike illness in babies. There appears to be some cross relationship between this virus and mumps. Children who have been infected with types 1 and 3 parainfluenza usually have a mild illness, but occasionally the viruses may be responsible for various forms of bronchitis and pneumonia. Crouplike symptoms have been associated with all of the first three types. They probably represent the most important *known* cause of croup among infants and children. The role of type 4 is not as yet clearly defined, although rarely it is responsible for sending a child to the hospital.

These viruses tend to cause epidemics particularly in closed populations such as orphanages, but it is believed that the agents will cause sporadic disease, as they are readily found almost any time of the year. They also have a tendency to cause disease early in life, as most children have antibodies by the time they are ready to go to school. The first infection is often more severe with fever, and as many as one third of the children may have various forms of pneumonia. The infection rate in the adult is lower primarily because most adults have antibodies (as pointed out in the volunteer study), particularly in captive groups in close proximity to each other.

To close the discussion of the parainfluenza agents, first cousins of influenza, mention should be made of two or three additional virus diseases which belong in this same large family. The first of these is Newcastle disease, which causes a mild inflammation of the eyes especially in individuals who work with infected chickens. The virus that is responsible for various forms of mumps, including mumps encephalitis, is also a part of this particular group. It now appears that the measles virus and related agents will eventually be classified as myxoviruses. The parainfluenza viruses are the most important causes of croup. They are reported to be responsible for 7 to 16 per cent of all respiratory illnesses in children.

■

Another myxovirus called respiratory syncytial (RS) was first discovered in chimpanzees with colds, but it was not long before it was found that it was the most common cause of serious respiratory illnesses in young infants. Its seriousness for infants cannot be overemphasized, as it appears to cause epidemics annually, particularly in nurseries or isolated groups of infants and young children. In adults, on the other hand, it has been found in relation to mild illnesses or colds, and again like parainfluenza it may cause illness even in the presence of antibodies.

In tissue culture the virus causes small masses to appear in cells called inclusion bodies. These bodies are found usually as round structures in the outer part of the cell and not in the core or nucleus (see accompanying picture, Figure 7). Similar bodies were found by the writer in the lungs of infants some 25 years ago in association with an epidemic of acute respiratory disease in an orphan home for infants. The symptoms of the babies in that epidemic were similar in all respects to those recently reported as due to RS viruses. Symptoms varied from the mild cases presenting cough and sneezing, only with little or no fever, to infants in whom the lungs were involved, with serious disease and occasionally a fatal outcome.

Inclusion bodies, which are uniformly present in virus cultures, may be found in the lungs of fatal cases. It is

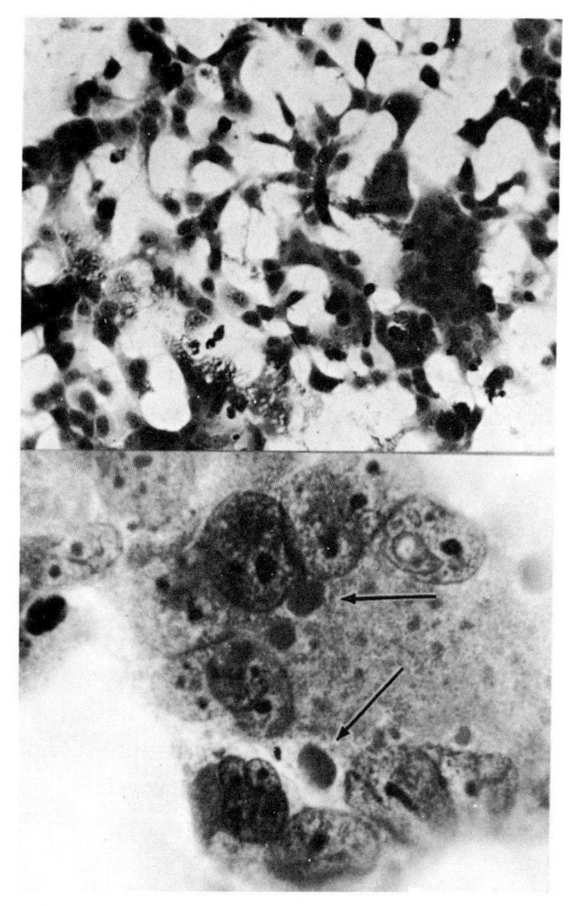

*Figure 7. The upper figure is a microscopic picture of the respiratory syncytial virus growing in tissue culture. The lower figure is an enlargement, and the arrows point to virus inclusion bodies in the outer part of the cell. By permission of the* Journal of the American Medical Association.

important to keep in mind that the so-called newer virus diseases are not really new, but are only newly discovered. While serious and sometimes fatal in infants, it is now recognized as an infection that occurs in older children and adults and is usually mild with all the features of the common cold.

■

Work is progressing in the research laboratories toward the development of a vaccine for the parainfluenza and RS viruses. Their prevalence must be critically assessed in order to determine the importance and need for a vaccine. These viruses are extremely significant and may cause fatal disease in infancy and early childhood. Serious consideration for an effective vaccine in this age group is of real importance. The role of these vaccines in adult illnesses is minimal, and except under rare circumstances a vaccine probably would not be generally employed. The greater stability of the parainfluenza viruses as compared to influenza would suggest that vaccines might be even more effective. It has recently been found that RS virus is "highly unstable and grows poorly in tissue culture." The problem of an effective vaccine remains to be solved.

To conclude, the parainfluenza or croup viruses and the RS viruses cause a wide spectrum of illness with the serious forms occurring most commonly in infants and young children; whereas adults who are infected usually have a mild, coldlike illness. Work on vaccines to prevent these diseases is progressing. A vaccine should be most worthwhile, particularly to protect infants. Nearly all adults have antibodies to parainfluenza and RS viruses. RS antibodies are transmitted to newborn babies, yet this virus is the most important cause of pneumonia in the first six months of life. This leaves the question of the protective effect of antibodies in doubt as far as RS virus is concerned. It is known that adults will develop colds caused by these viruses despite good levels of antibodies in their blood.

# 6 Adenovirus Infections and Their Prevention

These new viruses, discovered about ten years ago, are very important causes of coldlike illnesses in human beings. The discovery of the first viruses was made by growing pieces of tonsils that had been removed from children who seemed to be well at the time of operation. Peculiar changes took place in the cell cultures indicating that a virus might be present. It was found that cells grew out from the original fragments of tonsils, and in two to three weeks they formed clumps as a result of the injury caused by the hidden viruses which were living in the tonsils and adenoids. When the infected fluids were inoculated into fresh cultures of cells they again caused the destructive changes.

Soon these same viruses were discovered in military recruits and were shown to be commonly associated with coldlike illnesses. This disease was called ARD for Acute Respiratory Disease and was recognized as a throat infec-

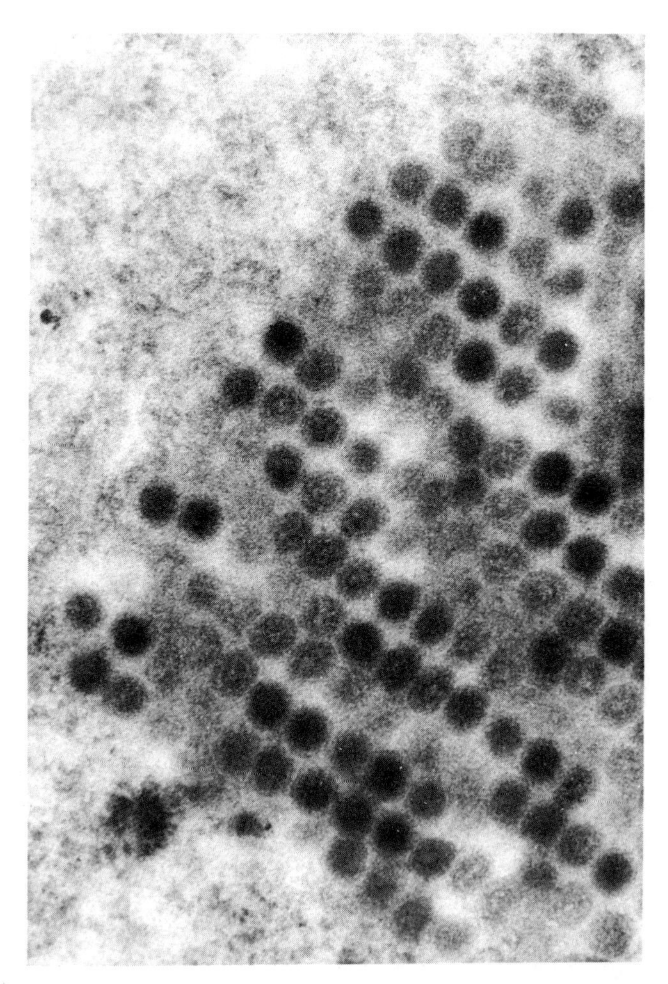

*Figure 8. An electron microscopic picture of adenoviruses, showing their arrangement in the form of a crystal. Magnified 120,000 times. From C. Morgan, C. Howe, H. M. Rose, and D. H. Moore, (1956): Structure and Development of Viruses Observed in the Electron Microscope. IV. Viruses of the RI–APC group,* J. Biophys. & Biochem. Cytol., *2:351. By permission of the Rockefeller Institute, 1956, New York, N.Y., Publisher, and by permission of The Macmillan Company,* Newer Virus Diseases.

tion not caused by bacteria such as "strep." There are now more than 30 distinct types of adenoviruses which have been found in human beings. The most common illness caused by these agents are acute tonsillitis and sore throat.

Certain types are known to be a frequent cause of epidemics among military recruits—type 4, in particular. It is rare in children. Type 8 is considered to be the cause of an epidemic eye disease known as keratoconjunctivitis. This disease is common in shipyard workers, particularly those who receive some injury to their eyes. Keratitis, inflammation of the surface of the eye, has been associated with several other types of adenoviruses as well.

As studies progress and our clinical knowledge is applied to this large group of viruses, it is apparent that the overlapping of symptoms and signs makes it almost impossible to attach anatomical terms such as tonsillitis to them. Distinguishing among the many numbered types becomes confusing and meaningless. It would appear practical and realistic to refer to these as adenovirus infections, with a full awareness of the wide range of symptoms and signs that are caused by these viruses. Acute tonsillitis with or without white spots in the throat is perhaps the most common form of adenovirus infection in children and often represents one of their earliest acute illnesses. It starts with a high fever and occasionally is accompanied by a convulsion.

Adenoviruses have been reported from many countries of the world and are recognized as causing illness in all age groups. A newborn baby usually has some protection or immunity, which he has acquired from his mother. The protection disappears in the early weeks and months of life and then is gradually acquired again as the baby gets these infections during childhood. More than half the infants tested between the ages of 6 and 12 months demonstrate protective substances in their blood (antibodies) to at least one of the adenoviruses. Further studies have indicated that infection spreads rapidly in the family, in summer camps, and in hospitals. Swimming pools are suspected as contributing to the spread of infection. The actual incidence of adenovirus infection varies a great deal in the civilian population, but it is known to be high among military recruits.

One of the first epidemics to be recognized as due to these viruses occurred in a children's camp in the summer of 1955. The campers had sore throats, and often spots were seen on the tonsils. The first wave of the epidemic was mild: fevers ranged from 100 to 101 degrees. No clear-cut diagnosis was made during this first wave, but in their report the doctors expressed concern as to whether or not they might be having a mild epidemic of poliomyelitis.

The second wave of illness began late in July and was more severe, involving over 60 per cent of the campers. This epidemic was featured by sore throat, headache, muscle aches, eye discomfort, and complaints of pain in the stomach. Many boys complained of stiffness and pain in the neck, back, and leg muscles, suggesting again a possible diagnosis of some kind of meningitis or polio. Inflammation in the eyes occurred in most of the patients, sometimes involving only one eye. The nose became obstructed and a discharge developed in several patients. The children also complained of earache, and evidence of infection in the ears was found in a third of them. Swelling of the glands in the neck was a common finding. Fever persisted for four or five days and often reached 104 degrees F. (40°C.). Although antibiotics were employed generously, no apparent effect was observed. Cultures for bacteria were uninformative, but adenovirus type 3 was isolated from the nose and throat of many of the campers.

An epidemic as severe and clear-cut as this in an isolated group of children would not ordinarily be confused or designated as a common cold. Yet it might well have been necessary to differentiate it from influenza, Coxsackie infections, streptococcal sore throats, poliomyelitis, and infectious mononucleosis. When any of these diseases occur in sporadic or mild form, they are often called colds.

The Commission of Acute Respiratory Diseases during the Second World War described clearly the features of ARD in military recruits. Records of blood samples taken from the soldiers over a ten-year period showed that adenoviruses were responsible for the disease. Cough and hoarseness, irritated throats, and nasal obstruction were the principal symptoms. The whole spectrum of illness was observed, from mild colds to severe, including a few cases of virus pneumonia.

Evidence of the spectrum is clearly demonstrated in new recruits in the army, where it is known that the majority (80 per cent) may suffer from an adenovirus infection within the first few months in service. One large study shows that about 20 per cent are sick enough to be admitted to the hospital with an acute illness; 15 per cent of these develop pneumonia. Forty per cent have an inapparent illness, as shown by blood tests, and continue about their normal activities.

A few reports in the recent medical literature have suggested a possible relationship of adenovirus infection with a disease called *roseola infantum.* This illness is most commonly seen in infants between the ages of 6 and 18 months, when they no longer have protective antibodies from their mothers. The babies have an unexplained fever followed by a rash usually after the fever goes away.

In a recent report from Helsinki, Finland, adenoviruses were isolated from several of their patients with a rash considered to be typical of roseola infantum. The symptoms were compared in the babies with the rash and those with a proved diagnosis of adenovirus infection. A striking degree of similarity between the two diseases was found. Further studies will undoubtedly clarify the possible relationship.

Vaccines for adenoviruses have been shown to provide protection against certain particular types, and in the military situation they have proved to be highly effective after a single inoculation. Their use in civilian populations has not received wide acceptance. Additional problems in production of the vaccine have arisen with respect to contaminating viruses that have been shown in animals to cause a cancerous change. It should be pointed out at once that their possible role in causing cancer in man has been entirely negative. Present regulations by the government for vaccine manufacture prohibit the presence of the contaminating virus in vaccines.

The first adenovirus types to be isolated have been most commonly associated with acute tonsillitis or sore throat in infants and children, but response to vaccines containing these types is notably less effective. It is difficult to protect against certain types commonly found in children when they have not had a previous experience with the infection. Consideration for vaccination by pills to be taken by mouth has been tried, because of the fact that these viruses persist throughout the bowel. So far, the results have been good, and the method holds real promise provided safety factors can be established. Successful trials among military recruits were reported in February 1966.

■

In summary, adenoviruses are common causes of acute respiratory disease in infants and children, producing acute tonsillitis frequently with white spots. They represent a most important cause of acute disease in new recruits in the army, among whom the spectrum of disease has been clearly established from inapparent illness to virus pneumonia. Oral vaccines are under intensive study and hold real promise of effective protection from attack by these common viruses. The illness should be called an adenovirus infection, not just tonsillitis or ARD. It is estimated that about 10 per cent of all acute respiratory illnesses seen in children's hospitals are due to adenoviruses.

# 7 About Measles (Rubeola)

Measles is one of the oldest and most important diseases of mankind. The first recognized accounts of measles are accredited to Rhazes (860–932). Although he distinguished between measles and smallpox, he thought the two conditions were related. This concept persisted into the eighteenth century, when Mead stated his opinion that "The measles has a great affinity with the smallpox."

The name "measles" is accredited to John of Gaddesden (1280–1361) as the equivalent of the Latin term *morbilli*. The English word is derived from the Latin *miselli*. Although measles was clearly differentiated from smallpox, it continued to be confused with scarlet fever, until Thomas Syndenham (1624–89) separated the two in his discourse on the measles epidemic in London in 1670. Syndenham quite clearly pointed out that coughs, sneezing, watering of the eyes, and sensitivity to light were distinct parts of measles. He described the eruption, which appeared on the fourth or fifth day on the forehead and the face and extended from there over the entire body. The rash then became rough and faded, leaving a fine, branlike scaling. Syndenham believed measles itself was not fatal but that the danger to life arose from other diseases which complicated measles, particularly pneumonia. He described a severe epidemic of measles in 1674, in which infants were heavily involved and the death rate was high due to lung complications. In 1662 measles was listed as the leading cause of death among children under six. However, it was not a dreaded disease. In 1785 Heberden stated: "The measles being usually attended with very little danger, it is not often that a physician is employed in this distemper." In 1762 Tissot stated that people rarely die of measles and when the outcome is fatal it is due to complications.

Epidemics in the New World were described as early as 1519 in Santo Domingo and 1531 in Mexico. An extremely severe outbreak occurred in Ecuador in 1785 in which more than 2,400 deaths occurred at Quito. Measles was recorded in epidemic form in New England shortly after the first settlements were established. An epidemic occurred in Boston and surrounding communities in 1657 and again in the winter of 1687–88. Epidemics of varied severity occurred throughout the colonies during the first half of the eighteenth century. The disease did not become endemic in the colonial period, and epidemics were usually followed by a period of relative immunity until a new population had appeared on the scene from immigration or new births.

Epidemiology in America was similar to that observed in the classic studies recorded by a young Danish physician, Peter Ludwig Panum, who visited the Faroe Islands in 1846. He was sent to study the epidemic which was occurring there after an interval of 65 years—the previous epidemic having occurred in 1781. The majority of the population of less than 8,000 people was involved. Over 6,100 patients were ill with measles, and 102 deaths resulted. Panum recorded many of the classic features of measles, including the incubation period of 13 to 14 days. He established the fact that immunity was lifelong. Individuals over 65 who presumably had had measles in 1781 did not get the disease. He pointed out the contagious nature of the disease, particularly early in its course.

The same complacency that exists today about measles and its severity existed then. A passage from Panum's thesis states: "The measles is a disease so generally familiar and so almost trivial that it might be supposed that observations in regard to it could offer nothing new except in special cases with more or less rare complications."

Attempts to transmit measles were carried out about the middle of the eighteenth century, when Francis Home reported the results of his studies. He carried out an experiment known as *morbilisation,* which was patterned after vaccination for smallpox. It was an attempt to produce a mild form of the disease to achieve immunity. Home induced several parents to permit their children to be inoculated with fresh blood from patients who were in the acute stage of the disease. The soaked pieces of cotton were placed on the skin over fresh cuts, or in the nose. Within a week seven children out of twelve came down with measles. Great hope prevailed for the prevention of this disease by a method similar to vaccination for smallpox. The practice was referred to as "the most powerful means of alleviating the common sequences of measles."

Measles was successfully transmitted to monkeys in 1898 and again in 1911. The virus was cultivated in tissue culture in 1938 and in chick embryos in 1940. The discovery that viruses would grow in tissue culture and produce destructive changes in the cells was made first in 1931. The practical application of this contribution was delayed another 20 years until antibiotics could be used to control bacterial contamination in the cultures. The classical studies with the polioviruses were followed almost immediately by the clear demonstration that measles virus when grown in test tubes produced very distinct changes. When a child recovers from measles, the serum part of his blood will prevent the changes in a test-tube culture of measles. This provides the proof and clear identification of the virus as being measles. Epidemics occur with a distinct periodicity about every two to five years in large centers of population. The disease tends to vary in its severity, which may be related to the secondary complicating bacteria present in the community. Bacteria have accounted for the high mortality in some past epidemics, but at the present time a very real mortality from measles per se is recognized, with over four hundred deaths a year in the United States. In some epidemic seasons as high as a hundred deaths in one month have been recorded. The rare complication of encephalitis remains by far the most serious problem that exists with measles today.

The age incidence appears to be lower in large urban centers, as most children come in contact with measles in the preschool years. In contrast, in rural communities children may escape measles until young adulthood. This was clearly evident in the First World War, at which time young men from the country were brought together into military camps and serious epidemics of measles occurred.

Many of the newly discovered viruses may cause rashes, which undoubtedly in the past have been confused with measles or which have been called second or third attacks; but the epidemic nature and the typical features of measles do not usually lead to confusion. A classical case of measles might be defined as a severe cold accompanied by a rash in two to five days following the onset of cough, running nose, and inflammation of the eyes. In addition to these classic early symptoms of measles, spots may occur inside the mouth called Koplik spots, first described in 1896.

In his book on air-borne infections, Dr. Dwight O'Hara states that measles is often diagnosed as a common cold until its true character is revealed by its later stages. Conversely, when definite exposure to measles is suspected, a common cold may be thought to be measles until it subsides without displaying the characteristic rash of this disease. He propounds the idea that a first attack of measles may be typical with a classic rash, and he then goes on to suggest that immunity may be maintained by mild or inapparent infections often passed off as colds. This, he states, may account for the lifelong immunity so commonly recognized in measles. This hypothesis has not as yet been proved. However, infection by the measles virus without rash has been reported. It has been successfully identified by finding the virus, particularly in association with other chronic debilitating illnesses such as leukemia and cystic fibrosis.

> In the H. family there were two children—a boy aged three and a girl aged eight. The doctor was called one morning because the mother thought the boy had some kind of rash, but when the visit was made a few hours later, there was no sign of either exanthem or enanthem [see glossary—J.M.A.]. There was no fever or other discernible sign of illness and the mother was apologetic for having been, as she thought, unduly apprehensive and perhaps imaginative about her child. There was measles at the time in the neighborhood and at the girl's school, but there had been no known exposure of the three-year old boy. No diagnosis could be made and the boy remained well; but twelve days later the older sister developed a florid attack of measles. The boy now slept with his measly sister and no attempt was made to keep them apart; the boy was surely exposed to measles, but he remained well! He had never before had measles, and has never contracted it since, although he was again exposed at a later date. What this careful mother had really observed was undoubtedly an attack of inapparent measles, an attack which her doctor could not diagnose, but which was nevertheless a contagious disease for the patient's sister and conferred a demonstrated immunity upon the patient himself.*

* Dwight O'Hara, M.D., *Air-Borne Infection: Some Observations on its Decline* (New York: The Commonwealth Fund, 1943).

The first symptoms appear in ten to twelve days and the rash almost exactly on the fourteenth day when a clear-cut exposure is well known. There are three recognized stages of the disease: the first is the incubation period and the second is the period prior to the rash, at which time spots appear in the mouth, usually seen best inside the cheeks opposite the molar teeth. The typical Koplik spot has a whitish-blue center with a little area of redness surrounding it. These spots may appear from one to four days prior to the onset of the rash (the second stage), which appears first on the face and body, subsequently spreading to the arms and hands with fading in the original areas. The rash is often blotchy in character and tends to be flat rather than raised. One of the typical and classic features of the measles rash is that it fades, leaving behind a brownish pigment with a fine, branlike peeling. The symptoms of cough, coryza, and conjunctivitis, the three C's of measles, tend to increase in severity, as does the fever, until the onset of the rash on the face and body. In the uncomplicated case this represents the height of illness, following which recovery may take place in a very few days.

Complications are marked by the continuing cough and fever, and signs of pneumonia may become evident. Pneumonia may be caused directly by the measles virus, and fatalities have been recorded in which no complicating bacteria have been found. The onset of encephalitis is marked by increasing fever, often higher than it was initially, and frequently accompanied by a convulsion. This rare complication of measles may be the first sign of illness, or it may occur at the height of the disease, but it usually makes its appearance from two to five days following the onset of the rash. Irritability and drowsiness are common symptoms, and profound coma may indicate encephalitis. These symptoms may persist for weeks, followed by complete recovery, but in as many as half of the cases of encephalitis, evidence of serious aftereffects are observed. Changes in the brain wave patterns in these patients are well recognized, and even in uncomplicated measles these changes may occur in surprisingly high incidence. Emphasis is placed on this serious feature in order to impress you with the importance of measles prevention. This is possible with safe and effective vaccines recently developed. Further details of the vaccine will be discussed later in this chapter.

Probably the disease that is most often confused with regular measles is rubella—the light, "three-day measles," sometimes called German measles—which may lack symptoms such as cough and running nose. These symptoms may be mild and associated with a slight throat irritation, but they are rarely if ever accompanied by pneumonia due to the rubella virus. Rubella is most serious when it occurs in pregnant mothers very early in their pregnancy. In known epidemics due to the rubella virus the unborn baby may be injured, and certain striking changes are clearly associated with this disease. The babies may be mentally retarded, may have cataracts in their eyes, or may have abnormalities of the heart. Deafness is also commonly associated with this condition.

Rubella or German measles has been known to occur without a rash, and it is therefore possible that many young adults are immune to rubella who have had no knowledge of the illness. There are several other virus diseases in which a blotchy, measly-like rash must be considered. These include the ECHO viruses, rarely Coxsackie viruses, and a disease known as roseola infantum. The latter may on occasion be important to consider in arriving at a correct diagnosis. Efforts have been made to compare roseola infantum and adenovirus infections in which a rash may occur in approximately one fifth of the infants having an illness caused by adenovirus (Chapter 6). The rash of roseola infantum tends to appear after the fever subsides and consequently is quite different from the rash of regular or common measles, which usually occurs at the height of the fever.

On March 21, 1963, an effective vaccine for regular measles was licensed and undoubtedly represents one of the great milestones in medical history. This was accomplished after many years of work on the part of many persons following the successful isolation of the measles virus in tissue culture by Drs. John Enders and Thomas Peeples. The virus was tamed and a weakened form of measles resulted, which made possible the early trials of the vaccine. Prior to licensing, extensive field trials were carried out over a period of several years, establishing the safety and efficacy of the vaccine.

Measles is a world-wide disease, and it respects no boundaries. In the United States there are over four hundred deaths per year, and in areas of the world where malnutrition and other disease such as tuberculosis are common, the death rate in children is extremely high. In 1960,

85,000 children died of measles in India, and in certain countries of Africa the mortality from measles in childhood is 25 to 50 per cent.

Although often considered a trivial and unimportant disease, even by members of the medical profession, the disease is extremely serious and the aftereffects may be damaging for life. There are approximately 4,000,000 cases of measles per year in the United States. The incidence of encephalitis varies, but it averages close to one per thousand reported cases in the United States. In virgin territories such as Greenland, the incidence has been recorded as high as six per thousand. The brain-damaging effects of this disease have been reported in more than 50 per cent of those afflicted. This could mean that as many as 2,000 children a year in this country may be brain injured as a result of measles.

These sobering thoughts should leave little doubt in our minds about the importance of vaccinating everyone who has not had regular measles. There are several vaccines available, the merits of which will be resolved by further careful study and observation over the next few years. Attenuated or tamed virus vaccines may produce fever, and some patients actually develop a rash, but these reactions are considerably less than those of the wild or natural disease. Immunity appears to be solid and long lasting. A killed vaccine is also available; it is less effective as an immunizing agent. The recommendations of your physician should be followed in the choice of the best vaccine for your child.

To summarize, regular or common measles (rubeola) is

an extremely important world-wide disease, characterized by cough, coryza, and conjunctivitis accompanied by a blotchy red rash. The virus may cause pneumonia by itself and rarely causes serious disease without a rash. A most important association, occurring about once in a thousand cases, is measles encephalitis, the precise cause of which is still unproved. Safe and effective vaccines for the prevention of measles are available and should be given to everyone who has not had regular measles. German measles (rubella) is an entirely different disease and is serious for the unborn baby when it attacks a mother early in her pregnancy. A vaccine against this virus disease is under intensive study. Early trials in 1966 have been successful in preventing rubella in human subjects.

# 8 Rhinoviruses and Human Volunteers in Research

This highly important and new group of viruses was defined following many years of research at the Harvard Common Cold Research Center located in Salisbury, England. After extensive research with common colds, a new technique of culturing the virus at lower temperatures, such as those that prevail at the surface inside the nose, was developed. Thus a whole new group of *rhino* or cold viruses was discovered. Similar or identical viruses were reported from the United States as responsible for the majority of common mild respiratory illnesses in adults. In children, the illness may be more serious. Several strains have been obtained from children with bronchitis or pneumonia. Researchers found that a special type of human cell culture called "diploid" greatly improved the ability to find viruses in patients with colds. The Harvard Hospital in Salisbury reported recently that they "can now isolate causative viruses from about 75% of patients with colds."

Many experiments were carried out to study how colds are transmitted from one person to another. The answer is not as simple as most people think, as it appears to be influenced by various seasonal and individual factors. We might ask: Do people actually sneeze virus? How long does virus persist in the air after being ejected by a cough or sneeze? Volunteers caught colds if they were in the same room as other subjects with colds and separated from them by blankets hung across the room. Sitting next to subjects with colds also permitted transmission; but when the virus was applied outside the nose or dried on a handkerchief, no colds were produced. It seemed obvious that the virus must land in some way inside the nose or on the surfaces of the eye in order to cause an illness.

Volunteers spent months on remote Scottish islands and failed to develop colds when given inoculations from the laboratory, but did develop colds when brought in contact with an individual imported from the mainland who had a naturally acquired cold. One of the difficult problems in the use of human volunteers is the uncertainty of the inoculation dose and of the way in which it produces a natural infection. The majority of the studies have been based on the spraying of suspensions of the virus into the nose and throat. Difficulties were overcome by designing experiments with small particle sprays. Very clear-cut results followed the accurate determination of the dose.

When individuals with high antibodies in their blood were sprayed with a certain dose of virus, they developed a running nose and nasal obstruction the following day, but the illness on the whole was very mild with no fever or change in the subject's antibodies. When volunteers with lower levels of antibodies were sprayed with the same dose, they had a longer incubation period of 2 to 3 days and a more severe illness with headache, sore throat, and chest pain. Illness appeared to be directly related to the amount of antibodies in the body prior to the inoculation. Several individuals with low antibodies actually developed spots of pneumonia, as shown by X ray.

A typical subject at the Common Cold Center in Salisbury receives his inoculation into the nose after four days of isolation. If successful, cough, sore throat, and coryza or running nose develop. The amount of nasal discharge is assessed by the use of paper handkerchiefs. The number is counted each day. The typical volunteer, who uses less than five in the preinoculation period, may use as many as 30 or more in a single day after onset of illness. Virus can be detected in the secretions from the nose on the second and third day, not by the fifth day; but a sample of blood obtained 14 days after innoculation showed a high rise in antibodies against the virus that was inoculated.

In a large group of human volunteers 16 developed colds, and 14 of these had little or no antibody at the time they were inoculated but did have significant rises of antibodies in the blood serum at 14 days. On the other hand, 33 volunteers developed no colds, and 26 of these were shown to have had a high antibody level at the time they received the inoculation. It was concluded that those individuals without antibodies developed colds and that those who had antibodies did not develop colds, thus demonstrating the clear protection afforded by previous experience with the virus. We do develop protective antibodies against colds.

The term "rhinovirus" was recently adopted by the International Committee for this rather large group of viruses, which classically seem to produce cough and running nose as the principal symptoms. Confusion exists, as it undoubtedly will for some time to come; many studies, particularly those in human volunteers, have shown that similar symptoms may be produced by many different viruses. Eighty or more rhinoviruses have been identified. Now that certain cold viruses are labeled, it is possible to control the dose and measure the antibody response of individuals who have colds. Antibody response may account for the fact that only 50 per cent of volunteers develop colds when exposed, and it has been shown that persons with antibodies may seem to be coming down with a cold, and then all symptoms will rapidly disappear. Undoubtedly this is an explanation of why many individuals swear by their "cold cure." When the first symptoms appear, the favorite remedy is taken—and the next day the "cold" is gone.

Chilling experiments with volunteers did not show any particular influence on susceptibility to colds. Some volunteers were given an inoculation followed by a hot bath and made to stand in a draft in wet bathing suits. Some took walks in the rain and sat around in wet clothes. Other subjects were given the same chilling treatments with inoculations which contained no virus. No significant differences were found in these various well-controlled groups, and it even turned out in a few experiments that virus inoculation plus chilling sometimes caused fewer colds than chilling alone.

An incubation period of two to three days, which was clearly demonstrated in the volunteer experiments, would argue against the *chill* playing an immediate role in the subject's illness. On the other hand, when coming down with a cold one might feel "chilly."

Effective prevention or treatment for many different types of colds is unknown. Mother Nature is still doing the best job by providing us with an assortment of antibodies, which tend to make our next cold mild or even inapparent. Getting older would appear to be the best protection against many of the common cold viruses which attack us. The problem is more serious in infancy, when colds may go on to pneumonia and death. Here the indications for vaccines are more clearly defined, and those now available should be used whenever advised. The importance of this problem in infancy will be discussed in more detail in the chapter concerned with sudden unexpected death in infants (Chapter XII).

The duration of immunity to common colds is poorly understood. Studies in Spitzbergen showed that 75 per cent of the winter residents acquired an acute respiratory disease within 30 days after the arrival of the first boat in the spring, and 90 per cent of the population experienced at least one cold during the shipping season. The natives also had many colds during the short summer season, and the interval of second attacks varied from three to seven weeks. An important question at this point would be: Is this a recurrence of the previous acute illness caused by the *same* germ or virus, or is it a visitation of a *new* and different type, one of a hundred or more which might have come into their environment?

Further studies with volunteers, employing nasal discharges collected from persons with colds, revealed that about half of the volunteers receiving the material developed colds. When this same material was mixed with human gamma globulin, colds occurred in only one-fifth as many subjects as those who did not receive the antibodies.

In an early volunteer study done in 1946, medical students were observed during an entire winter season with emphasis primarily on the *incidence* of colds following the use of concentrated gamma globulin. Gamma globulin is the fraction or part of the blood serum where antibodies are stored. When separated and concentrated, it may be transferred to other individuals by an inoculation. Prior to the time when many different causes of colds were known, it seemed worthwhile to see whether rather large amounts of antibodies, given regularly to human beings, would prevent or lessen the incidence of these common illnesses. A group of 70 medical students was divided equally according to their past experiences with colds. Large doses of gamma globulin were given to one group during the winter season at monthly intervals. Each of the 35 experimental subjects received nearly an ounce (30cc.) of this potent antibody material. The actual incidence of illness was reduced by 40 per cent in the experimental subjects, when compared with an equal number of their classmates who were living in the same environment during their first year in medical school. An evaluation of severity of illness likewise showed a significant reduction in the experimental subjects, particularly when compared with their previous seasons' experience.

Studies on protective serum antibodies have brought to light many long-sought-for answers regarding immunity to colds. Experiments involving human volunteers have shown that these common illnesses do cause an antibody response and partially protect the individual against reinfection. Antibodies developed slowly against many of these infectious secretions containing virus; serum collected a month after the initial infection had only slight protective powers. But serums collected 6 to 12 months after the infection showed almost complete protection against the infectious material that had produced the cold initially. After two years most of this protective capacity disappeared.

The conclusions that the researchers were able to draw from their studies suggested that the main preventive mechanism is directly related to antibodies. They concluded further that recovery from the initial infection appeared to be unrelated to the development of antibodies, and they mentioned that a nonspecific substance like interferon was more likely.

The many types of viruses that are now known to cause the mild illness that people call "colds" emphasize clearly that it is impossible to generalize regarding immunity. Research with volunteers has shown that illness may be produced in individuals with antibodies and the degree of protection is quite specific for the initial infection. Gamma globulin is *not* made up of nonspecific antibodies but contains very specific antibodies to *many different* viruses, several of which undoubtedly are still undiscovered. Its use is *not* recommended for the prevention of colds except in very special situations. Any protection afforded by gamma globulin is of rather short duration, as the effectiveness of this material lasts for only a few weeks when inoculated into human subjects. It is known as *passive* rather than the *active* protection; the latter type follows an acute infection.

Gamma globulin has been used to lessen the severity of an attack of measles, particularly during the incubation stage of the disease. If given early in relatively large amounts to a child exposed to measles, it might result in complete protection, but this only lasts for a few weeks and is not recommended in general as another exposure to measles may be unknown to the patient. If a shot of gamma globulin gave complete protection against a known exposure, it should be followed up in a month or two by active immunization against measles (Chapter 7).

What can be said about the value of masks in preventing the spread of colds or protecting the wearer from catching a cold? On the streets of Tokyo masks are a common sight: children in school play yards and even a taxi driver who has a cold might wear masks. There is no question that the germs that cause colds, viruses mainly, are spread in the air. Several types of masks have been designed to stop the droplets of the cough and sneeze. The most effective are composed of several layers of gauze, sometimes with a layer of cellophane in between. The really good mask is not worn for very long, for after it becomes saturated its effectiveness is gone. Researchers have studied the problem critically and find little or no value to the wearer. Sir Christopher Andrewes states, "Gauze masks worn by people with colds could well cause congestion, hinder air-flow and do the sufferer no good at all." One cannot help admiring the spirit of the wearer, who does not want you to "catch his awful cold." The masks do serve to warn others of the culprit.

In summary, the rhinoviruses were discovered and defined only recently, following the idea that they might grow best in tissue cell culture if the conditions found in the nose were simulated—that is, reduced temperatures and controlled acidity. They cause colds with cough, sneezing, and running nose in adults, as shown repeatedly in human volunteer experiments. They may cause more serious disease in infants and children. The difficulty lies in the large number of viruses, which are quite different and produce antibodies for themselves only. The many specific types help to explain the commonness of colds. Even if an adult has had many colds in the past, there may be a new one lurking on the doorstep or on the lips of a friend. There are more than 80 types of rhinoviruses identified and possibly many more to come. Their newness prevents any more detailed discussion, as there is still much to be learned about them. They are *not* the only cause of "colds" in man.

# 9 Polioviruses and Closely Related Viruses and "Summer Colds"

*Then came the tragic years that Eleanor Roosevelt recalls her "trial by fire." Her husband's illness—first diagnosed as a cold—turned out to be infantile paralysis.*

—from a newspaper account

Dr. Robert J. Huebner, a world authority on respiratory diseases and Director of the Virus Laboratories in the National Institutes of Health, states that "most infections with poliovirus are expressed simply as febrile pharyngitis or as 'summer colds.'" Mild infections caused by poliovirus cannot be distinguished from many other viruses now known to cause colds.

The large family of enteroviruses, more than 60 in number, includes the polioviruses, the Coxsackie viruses, and the new ECHO (enteric cytopathogenic human orphans) viruses. These agents have been called enteroviruses because they live and multiply in the intestinal tract. This large group is included under the picornaviruses, which also includes the rhinoviruses discussed in the previous chapter. The enteroviruses will be reviewed separately, although the features of these diseases all overlap, and the symptoms and spinal fluid findings are almost identical in all of them. There are, however, certain signs which tend to distinguish these diseases, particularly the incidence of paralysis, which is much more common in poliomyelitis.

The clinical features of these diseases are extremely varied. In order to understand the spectrum, it will be necessary to become acquainted with the entire symptom picture. One of the prime objectives of this book is to emphasize that a certain virus may cause simple colds and the *same* virus may cause a serious complication like encephalitis. The so-called "nuisance" or trivial illnesses always have the potential of becoming serious, and inflammation of the brain and heart have both been identified with many of the enteroviruses.

Until recently, little attention was paid to the possibility that the polioviruses may cause disease outside of the central nervous system. However, it is quite clear that these viruses, which are widely distributed throughout the world, may produce an illness that does not involve the nervous system. Following the severe epidemic that occurred in Minnesota in 1946, it was apparent that acute sore throat may be one of the chief complaints in patients with poliomyelitis. A group in Cleveland, Ohio, studying common illnesses reported family epidemics of poliomyelitis and "devil's grippe" (pleurodynia) in their search for the causes of acute respiratory illnesses. Four families were suffering from an acute sickness which they called "grippe." The poliovirus was identified in three of these families, and in the fourth the Coxsackie virus was found to be responsible for the acute illness. Blood tests in these families for the presence of antibodies clearly incriminated the viruses, which were isolated at the time of the acute illness.

Poliovirus was found in an epidemic in an institution in Germany in which the children became ill with mild fever and red throats. The epidemic spread rapidly and involved 26 patients; most were in the infant age group. The doctors described their patients as having acute rhinopharyngitis or running nose. Virus studies indicated that the poliovirus type 2 was responsible for the epidemic. Occasionally adenovirus infections have simulated poliomyelitis (Chapter VI).

In 1949 Dr. Gilbert Dalldorf reported on the isolation of a new virus he had found in children who were thought to have poliomyelitis. Patients were first discovered in Coxsackie, New York, and the Coxsackie viruses have continued to retain this name, for which the town is now famous. Since their discovery they have been identified in all parts of the world in association with many different types of illness. They represent another large family of viruses; 29 distinct types have been divided into two groups, A and B. Dr. Dalldorf inoculated newborn mice with specimens from the original children and found that the mice became ill and paralyzed. This does not happen when poliovirus is put into newborn mice, so it appeared likely to him that a virus different from polio was related to the illness of the children. The A type of virus commonly causes an illness with fever during the summer months. Patients complain of headache and occasionally stiffness of the neck and muscle soreness. Small blisterlike lesions appear in the throat, which later may ulcerate. Coxsackie

A viruses occasionally cause a rash, that may resemble chicken pox but that disappears quickly without leaving a crust or scar.

There are six different viruses in the B group, which are characterized by sudden high fever with severe chest pains sometimes referred to as "devil's grippe" or Bornholm disease. A few well individuals have been found to harbor the Coxsackie agents. The incubation period varies from four to five days, as studied in family groups, but reports indicate that these viruses cause acute sore throats without the blister formation and may be associated with general aching, some redness of the throat, chest pains, and chills.

A report from the Children's Hospital in Washington, D.C., recorded that a few patients have convulsions, but the majority complain of sore throat and difficulty in swallowing. Most characteristically, however, the little blisters appear on the back of the throat and tonsils. Since the advent of the polio vaccine these cases have assumed greater importance because paralysis may rarely be related to Coxsackie or other agents rather than failure of polio vaccination.

Acute inflammation of the heart is also a feature of the Coxsackie B infections, first discovered in newborn babies. This is a very serious illness when it occurs in infancy. It may cause a collapse of the heart, with a large liver and blueness, commonly ending fatally.

The advent of the tissue culture era resulted in the explosive discovery of many strange new viruses found in the stool specimens from individuals who were thought to be suffering from poliomyelitis. These viruses, which cause destruction of cells in tissue culture, were named Enteric Cytopathogenic Human Orphans (ECHO) because they were unassociated with a disease. The term ECHO was adopted with the idea that they would soon acquire other names, but ECHO has stuck, and more than 30 distinct types have now been identified. They cause a variety of grippelike or coldlike illnesses with fever and are frequently associated with acute diarrhea in infants. Some of the varieties cause a transitory infection of the intestinal tract, but are not considered lifelong residents like the colon bacteria commonly found there. The echoviruses may occur in the bowels of healthy children, particularly during the summer months, and are commonly found in large families of low incomes.

Certain types have a tendency to cause a coldlike illness which may occur during the cooler months of the year. One group studied in an orphanage in Washington, D.C., was clearly identified as causing mild colds only. The primary features were fever, running nose, mild redness of the throat and ears, as well as abnormal bowel movements. There may be slight fever for a day or two, associated with running nose, sneezing, and irritability. Cough also is a striking symptom. The spectrum of illness is very bizarre as a result of infection by these viruses.

Summer diarrhea may be a consequence of transitory infection with a large variety of bacteria, viruses, or both. Infections spread rapidly in families or communities, and the illness is rarely severe as indicated by the epidemic in Milwaukee, Wisconsin, in which 45,000 of the 750,000 inhabitants were ill with a similar illness caused by an echovirus. Only 149 cases were hospitalized. Surveys among children reveal that the incidence of these viruses is three to six times higher in children in the poorer districts of the city.

A disease originally described as Boston exanthem is known to be due to type 16 echovirus. The incubation period is four to five days, and fever may range from 101 to 104 degrees F. (38°C.–40°C.), lasting one to two days in patients who have signs of meningitis. Echovirus 9 may cause a rash similar to measles. It is most common in children, occurring in about 50 per cent of those infected. Rarely paralysis may occur. This virus may also cause fever and other signs of acute illness such as sore throat, sore eyes, and swelling of the glands in the neck. It is clear that the echoviruses cause illness in human beings, characterized by diarrhea in some patients as well as signs of a cold, sometimes associated with rash.

In 1956 a virus named JH was isolated from adults and children suffering from running nose and mild sore throat with a slight fever. At about the same time a virus known as "2060" was isolated among naval recruits with mild, coldlike illnesses. It appears that these two viruses are very similar, and they have both been identified as echovirus type 28. The problem of naming virus diseases is a difficult one, particularly when new viruses without a disease are being discovered almost daily. Several previously described diseases are gradually being identified as related to certain of the newly discovered agents.

Dr. Stuart-Harris in his 1960 review entitled "The Viruses of Human Disease" recognized the complex and unpredictable behavior of many new viruses and aptly stated, "it is perhaps fortunate that we do not have different illnesses to correspond with so many different viruses."

The Committee on the Control of Infectious Diseases of the American Academy of Pediatrics recommends that all children and young adults be immunized against poliomyelitis, the paralytic forms of which may thus be prevented. There are two available vaccines: the first is a killed vaccine (Salk) which must be injected, and the second is a weakened live vaccine (Sabin) which is taken by mouth. Both are licensed by the Public Health Service and have been given to millions of children and adults. Both vaccines have been effective in preventing paralytic poliomyelitis.

A critical evaluation of the virtues and limitations of each reveal a superiority for the oral preparation because of the ease with which it may be given, its ability to produce antibodies that last for a long time, and the possibility that polio may be eradicated by its use. A committee of the Academy recommends it for community-wide vaccination programs of children and young adults and for routine immunization in infancy.

There are certain warnings that should be kept in mind. The first is that the oral preparation should not be given within one month of other live vaccines such as measles and smallpox. Further, it is recommended that in order to avoid coincident infection by enteroviruses, which are most common in the summer months, a vaccination program should not be held during the natural polio season.

An exception would be the occurrence of an epidemic in a community, at which time vaccination with the *same* type of virus is recommended. Polio vaccine may be given at the time of the diphtheria-tetanus-pertussis (DPT) vaccine in young infants, followed a year later by a single booster dose of a preparation containing all three polioviruses. The injectable killed vaccine calls for four inoculations, three of which may be given at the time of the three DPT injections in young infants and the fourth at about fifteen months of age. Booster shots are recommended every two years for the time being. Finally, it should be stated that either the oral or injectable vaccine may be ineffective if the series is not completed.

In summary, enteroviruses live and grow in the intestines. There are more than 60 types, which include polio, Coxsackie, and echoviruses. They are known to cause varying degrees of encephalitis and occasionally paralysis, but several types also cause acute respiratory illnesses, "colds" which may or may not be associated with diarrhea. Two kinds of polio vaccines are available and will prevent paralysis due to the three polioviruses.

# 10 Primary Atypical Pneumonia and Virus Pneumonias

When the sulfa drugs and antibiotics such as penicillin came to be used widely for the treatment of pneumonia it was soon apparent that many patients failed to respond. The terms "atypical pneumonia" and "virus pneumonia" became the popular labels for such illnesses. There are many different kinds of pneumonia, and a list would include most of the diseases under discussion in this book. When seen as individual cases, the diagnosis may be most difficult, and the following diseases should be considered: influenza, measles, chicken pox, lymphocytic choriomeningitis, the bird pneumonias known as psittacosis or ornithosis, the adenoviruses, parainfluenzas, and some of the enteroviruses. The agents that cause these pneumonias do so on rare occasions only, and all of them may be responsible for mild, coldlike illnesses and probably cause inapparent infections most commonly.

Primary atypical pneumonia is a diagnosis that became

popular during the Second World War, when a distinct type of lung infection was recognized in our military camps and in certain colleges and other institutions. A great deal of confusion resulted, and primary atypical pneumonia was considered for many years to be caused by a virus.

Dr. Monroe Eaton and his associates in 1944 reported on a new agent they had found in a patient with atypical pneumonia. It caused an infection in cotton rats and hamsters as well as chick embryos. The serum from patients who recovered was capable of neutralizing Eaton's agent and in addition sometimes caused human blood cells to clump together, particularly when stored in the refrigerator. This property of serum is known as "cold agglutinin" and served for many years to separate primary atypical pneumonia from other atypical or virus pneumonias.

Secretions from patients with primary atypical pneumonia when inoculated into volunteers produced an illness in approximately 75 per cent of the subjects. A rise in cold agglutinin levels in many of the volunteers occurred in mild cases as well as in those with pneumonia.

The causative agent of this kind of pneumonia with cold agglutinins is a bacterium called *mycoplasma pneumoniae* (Eaton agent), the smallest free-living organism. It is a common cause of acute, coldlike illness, particularly in teen-agers and young adults. Following the discovery of the relationship of the Eaton agent and methods for detecting antibodies in the serum, it was learned that pneumonia occurs in only about one out of 30 individuals infected. The entire spectrum of illness including inapparent infection occurs as a result of infection by this little bacterium. Human volunteer studies have shown that reinfection may occur, but it is usually mild in the presence of antibodies. Rarely a type of meningitis may be associated with the mycoplasma germ. About 45 per cent of individuals infected with Eaton agent have a positive test for cold agglutinins in their serum. This phenomenon occurs in less than 10 per cent of pneumonia caused by viruses.

Eaton-agent pneumonia was found to occur in a high incidence among military recruits studied on Parris Island, South Carolina. An unusual opportunity was afforded to evaluate proved cases of atypical pneumonia and to compare them with similar pneumonias known to be due to viruses. Eaton-agent pneumonia may be successfully treated with antibiotics, so it is important to determine if this type of pneumonia is causing the patient's illness and to begin treatment early.

Pneumonia caused by the Eaton agent represents the far end of the spectrum and may be considered relatively uncommon. It is of interest, however, to note the low incidence of complications in this study of proved pneumonias that were *not* treated with antibiotics. One patient developed an encephalitis associated with Eaton-agent pneumonia. Intermittently the patient appeared confused and disoriented with aggressive behavior. After five weeks improvement occurred, and subsequently he made an uneventful recovery.

The early diagnosis of atypical pneumonia is still a difficult task from the signs and symptoms alone. The use of serum tests is dependent on the rise in antibodies in the blood, and this does not occur early in the illness. Patients who develop cold agglutinins (45 per cent of those known to be due to the Eaton agent) did experience a more severe illness, and the X-ray changes in the chest persisted longer. When the diagnosis of pneumonia was established, the course of illness tended to be prolonged, with 25 per cent of the patients having symptoms after four weeks. The acute symptoms of fever and headache were relieved between the third and tenth day, but the chest findings often persisted for several weeks.

# 11 Infectious Mononucleosis, Acute Infectious Lymphocytosis, and Lymphocytic Choriomeningitis

All three of these diseases have their puzzling features, and all of them need be considered in making a precise diagnosis of an acute respiratory illness. The cause of the first two is still unknown, and, although it is often presumed to be viral, little or no evidence exists for this theory. Lymphocytic choriomeningitis is caused by the virus of the same name. Certain symptoms are distinctive, and these will be related for each of these diseases.

Infectious mononucleosis (IM) or glandular fever implies that certain cells (monocytes) in the blood are involved in this disease, although this is not the case. The main disturbance is with the blood lymphocytes. Often considered a blood disease, the most striking features of infectious mononucleosis are fever with sore throat and swollen glands in the neck. It is obvious that this disease must be considered in diagnosing the various forms of tonsillitis. Epidemics have been reported, but the disease is not readily transmitted from one person to another. Colonel Hoagland's classic reports, based on his study over the years of cadets at West Point, show that although these young men live three to a room, he has failed to detect this disease in roommates. The incubation period is considered to be approximately eleven days, with some variability.

Although the glands in the neck predominate, there may be an increase in the size of the lymph nodes over the entire body. The spleen, which is a lymphatic organ, is increased in size and may be enlarged in about half of the cases. Occasionally a rash appears on the body between the fourth and tenth day. This is not a common occurrence, but it may complicate the diagnosis by adding one more rash disease to be eliminated. The liver frequently is tender and enlarged, and the patient may be yellow colored (jaundiced). Hepatitis is commonly associated with this condition. Blood serum tests indicating involvement of the liver are often abnormal and may remain so for a long period of time.

Infectious mononucleosis is very rarely associated with inflammation of the brain, but when it is, the common symptoms are headache, blurring of vision, mental confusion, and occasionally convulsions. An important complication is involvement of the heart, which is indicated by fever, general discomfort, and pain in the chest and shoulders. Electrocardiographic changes have shown acute inflammation of the coverings of the heart. One of the rare but serious aspects is the enlarged spleen, which has been reported to rupture and result in a fatality. A nineteen-year-old girl succumbed following the rupture of her spleen. At post-mortem examination many lymphocytic cells were found in the heart muscle, an indication of acute carditis. In cases with splenic enlargement great care should be exercised to protect this organ from any unusual stress or strain, including too vigorous examination by the doctor.

The diagnosis of this disease, the cause of which is unknown, rests largely on two important features. The first has to do with the abnormal lymphocytes in the blood, and the second with a test called the "heterophil antibody response." Lymphocytes are usually increased in number compared to the other cells and may be as high as 60 to 90 percent of the total. The heterophil antibodies, just referred to, appear during the first week of illness, and it is very helpful in making the diagnosis when they are found to be positive. There are a few other conditions in which a positive test may occur infrequently, including primary atypical pneumonia discussed in the previous chapter.

Colonel Hoagland emphasizes that 70 per cent of his patients complained of sore throat. He further points out that 100 per cent of the patients had enlarged lymph glands and that more than 80 per cent had inflammation of the tonsils. Puffy eyelids was a striking finding in the West Point cases, occurring in a third of the cadets. None of the patients reported by him had a rash.

The outlook for recovery is good even when the brain and liver have been involved. Rarely the disease may persist, with weakness and fatigue lasting for weeks and sometimes for months. Bed rest is considered important in the acute stages of the disease. No specific treatment is known, but it is important to keep a careful watch for complications.

■

Acute infectious lymphocytosis was considered to be closely related to infectious mononucleosis until certain distinct differences were revealed which clearly separated the two diseases. This disease is characterized by a marked increase in the number of lymphocytes in the blood, and because of the mild nature of the illness it may be the only finding. Fever and signs of a cold, occasionally with abdominal complaints, skin rash, and encephalitis, are the reasons why it has been confused with infectious mononucleosis. An entire family of six children was diagnosed as having acute infectious lymphocytosis on the basis of the great increase in lymphocytes in their blood. They were suffering from an illness which all agreed were "colds."

Epidemics have been described in institutions as well as families, with a tendency to involve the children. It is a mild disease, the most severe symptoms consisting of sore throat, vomiting, irritability, sometimes pain in the stomach, and occasionally diarrhea. Rashes and signs of encephalitis have rarely been reported. By far the commonest symptoms are those related to the nasal passages and the presence of a high white blood cell count, averaging 40,000 to 50,000 and rarely reaching as high as 100,000 per cubic millimeter. The lymphocytic cells, however, are not considered abnormal. This would tend to eliminate infectious mononucleosis at once, but it must also be differentiated from leukemia, whooping cough, and possible other rare conditions in which the lymphocytes may be increased. The white blood counts in whooping cough may occasionally be very high, but this disease is usually much more severe. No deaths have been reported from acute infectious lymphocytosis; no treatment is indicated, and the outlook is uniformly favorable.

■

The third disease, lymphocytic choriomeningitis, is included because there is evidence that this virus disease may cause acute, coldlike illnesses. The virus received its name because research with experimental animals showed that it produced inflammation in certain cells of the brain. Blood tests performed in the general population showed that many individuals have antibodies against this virus. This was particularly true if a history of a recent cold was obtained. The virus has been found to occur in certain common household animals, such as the mouse and the dog. It has been found in secretions from their noses as well as in the urine. Information on the natural history of this disease is extremely scanty, but it has produced a grippelike illness in laboratory workers, in whom it may be extremely serious.

One report in the literature records a laboratory worker who became ill with fever, general aches, sore throat, vomiting, cough, and a low blood count. The illness continued until the patient died, at which time there were no signs of meningitis or encephalitis. However, the lungs revealed pneumonia, and these same lymphocytic cells were involved in the inflammation. Virus was isolated from the blood and from *brain* tissues. A second patient, who assisted at the post-mortem examination of the first case, eight days later developed fever with a low white count and sore throat. Signs of acute respiratory disease progressed until, seventeen days later, with a persistent sore throat and pneumonia, he died. Lymphocytic choriomeningitis virus was again isolated from the lung tissues. Although not a common cause of acute respiratory disease, certainly lymphocytic choriomeningitis must rarely be considered among the many known causes of colds.

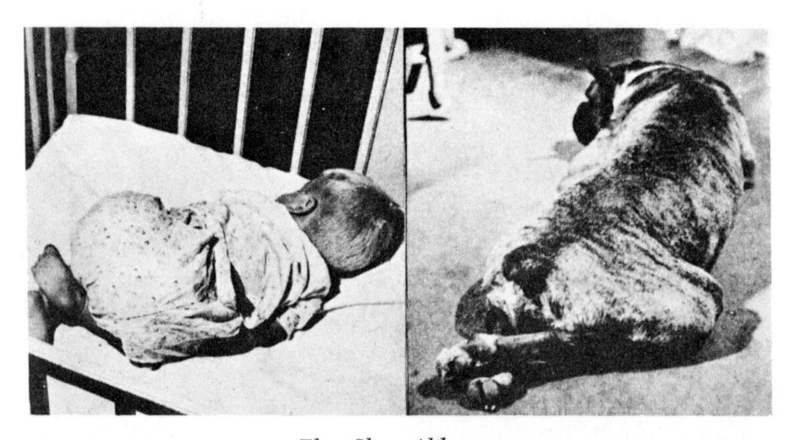

*They Sleep Alike*
*Animals and human beings have much in common*
*Reprinted with the permission of* Minneapolis Star Journal

# 12 Sudden Unexpected Death in Infants

From the Santa Monica, California, *Evening Outlook*, January 23, 1953:

> A disease, not yet positively identified, but which starts much like a common cold and then kills its infant victims within a few hours, claimed its *sixth* victim in Tacoma, Washington, yesterday. The latest fatality was three-month-old David [L.]. Mr. and Mrs. [L.] said their child caught what they thought was a slight cold Wednesday. They were not alarmed, but when they awoke yesterday the child was dead. Five other children have died in the same manner after contracting what appeared to be mild infections that did not even lead the parents to take the children's temperatures. The County coroner said an autopsy indicated that Baby [L.] died of a pneumonic virus. He compared the symptoms of the disease to those of the severe influenza epidemic which killed so many Americans during World War I.

These tragic events have the medical profession baffled. The mystery persists in spite of intensive research into the causes of sudden unexpected death in infants. This descriptive diagnosis requires further definition, as the condition represents a specific condition and should be designated as such in order to focus sharply on the basic problem. Deaths do occur suddenly, usually while the baby is unattended in his crib, but a careful history often reveals that the baby has been having mild symptoms sometimes consisting of sneezing, stuffy nose, or mild diarrhea. These symptoms as a rule are unassociated with fever or other signs of illness and do not disturb the family unduly. Many of these babies have been seen by their doctor a few hours or a day before the tragic event, or their mother has talked with the doctor on the telephone about the baby's mild illness. This is the reason why the word "unexpected" is commonly employed in discussions of this problem. These apparently mild illnesses may be very significant, and this is the primary reason why the condition is included in a book on common respiratory illnesses.

There is a definite and characteristic age period when sudden deaths occur. It is mainly from one to six months, rarely occurring prior to one month or six weeks of age and quite uncommon after six months, but these deaths may occur up to one or two years of age. This specific period is considered significant, as it relates to the problem of immunity or *lack of immunity* on the part of the baby to many of the very common illnesses which he is about to experience for the *first* time in his life.

Nature has provided the newborn baby with many antibodies from his mother, but these are transferred to the baby in direct proportion to the level existing in the mother's blood. They are highly significant in the case of poliomyelitis, measles, and mumps, but on the other hand small amounts or none may be transferred against many of the common respiratory viruses. They are often dissipated or lost in the first few weeks or months of life. In this period there is a great risk that the baby may get certain common infections. In addition to this risk, the baby has relatively small lungs. Like his hand, his lung is there in all its parts, but it is small. When the main job of ventilation is seriously compromised, swelling and congestion occur in the pulmonary tree. This can lead to a critical lack of oxygen, which may represent the primary cause of the baby's death.

The baby that is born prematurely receives a smaller supply of antibodies from its mother, as most of these protective substances cross over to the baby during the last two months before birth. Babies born with an abnormality in their hearts also are at a handicap, particulary when they are confronted with their first cold. The incidence of crib deaths is twice as high in babies who are born prematurely or who have a congenital heart condition.

Other obvious causes which may be discovered at post-mortem are blood poisoning with bacteria in the blood and occasionally meningitis. These conditions undoubtedly cause the baby's death, but it is important to remember that it may have been started off by a primary illness involving the respiratory passages which allowed bacteria to get into the blood or into the coverings of the brain. The majority of the post-mortem studies do show congestion and signs of inflammation in the pulmonary tree, but there are many cases in which these signs are minimal or appear insufficient to account for death. However, their presence in the *majority* of cases must be taken seriously and the causes of pulmonary disease considered and weighed carefully among the possible causes of these tragic deaths.

Many theories have been proposed—perhaps the oldest and most discredited theory is that these babies smother in their beds. Along the same lines, doctors have suggested that obstruction to the breathing passages was caused by choking on vomitus or by the swelling of the thymus gland. However, evidence, found in the lungs of these babies will not support the diagnosis of asphyxia, in which the lungs are often pale rather than congested. The latter is the common finding in association with sudden deaths. The complete lack of antibodies in the blood has not been proved, but, as pointed out earlier, certain *specific* antibodies may be lacking owing to their failure to be transmitted from the mother in sufficient amounts. It is a fact that the blood serum level of gamma globulin, which is the substance where antibodies are located, is reduced by half in the first month of life. It remains low and gradually increases in the first six months, at which time the incidence of crib deaths drops sharply. We could say that the incidence of sudden unexpected death and the levels of gamma globulin in the babies' blood are just the opposite of each other—that is, when the crib deaths are highest, the babies' blood is at the lowest point with respect to antibodies or gamma globulin.

Several investigators have studied the problem of increased sensitivity to cow's milk. They suggest that a small amount of milk comes up from the stomach while the baby is asleep; it then is aspirated into the pulmonary passages, and this accounts for the massive congestion of the lungs. Babies who died unexpectedly have been studied to determine the amount of antibodies against milk in their blood, and critical results have shown that a certain proportion of these babies do have antibodies—but no more than other babies in this same age group who are perfectly well. Thirty-eight cases of crib death were studied for milk sensitivity; 14 of this small group had no detectable antibodies, and those who did fell within the normal range for babies at their respective ages.

Figures brought out at a conference on sudden death reveal that large numbers of deaths are still reported annually as related to "accidental mechanical suffocation." In one year this diagnosis was made on 1,663 infants, with an additional 929 infant deaths attributed to enlargement of the thymus gland. Another large group of over 4,000 infants was classified as "unknown cause of death." The problem is large and warrants most serious consideration and intensive research.

The story is usually a simple and uncomplicated one. The baby, often between the ages of two and five months (who may be having a mild cold), is suddenly discovered by a member of his family to be dead. In the excitement of finding the baby, the immediate circumstances are often not carefully observed. The first natural impulse is to consider that the baby has smothered. Unless a thorough post-mortem examination is carried out, this conclusion may be reported by the coroner as the cause of death.

Dr. Katherine Bain comments,

> The story does not end here. The parents develop a great sense of guilt which can disturb their own lives for years. Sometimes accusation of one parent about the carelessness of the other leads to quarrels and break-up of the home. Occasionally authorities, friends or neighbors may imply intentional neglect or even homicide. The social and emotional repercussions of such an "accident" are therefore widespread and of great importance.

At the conference on sudden death, the late Dr. Jacob Werne, a pathologist who devoted much of his life to the study of this problem, reported that "pulmonary congestion is almost invariable, and when extreme is often associated with extensive pleural hemorrhage." He placed great stress on the amount of extra fluid found in the lung. This excess fluid is often blood tinged and results in the diminished air content of the pulmonary tree.

In 1943 this writer reported three cases of sudden unexpected death related to pneumonia with evidence of hemorrhagic or bloody congestion of the lungs as the most outstanding finding. The type of cells found in the inflammation was similar to those that are frequently associated with viral rather than bacterial diseases. Although virus studies have been extremely unrewarding in the past, it is possible with newer methods that further discoveries will be forthcoming. A recent report revealed enteroviruses in 12 of 48 sudden-death infants studied in Cleveland, Ohio. It was pointed out earlier, in the chapter on poliomyelitis and related agents, that these viruses can cause acute inflammation of the lung.

An increased incidence of sudden crib death has occurred during influenza epidemics as reported in the Denver, Colorado, experience in October 1957 (Chapter IV). The death rate is definitely higher in the winter months coincident with the increased incidence of acute respiratory disease (see the accompanying graph from the Public Health Service, Figure 9). The most convincing

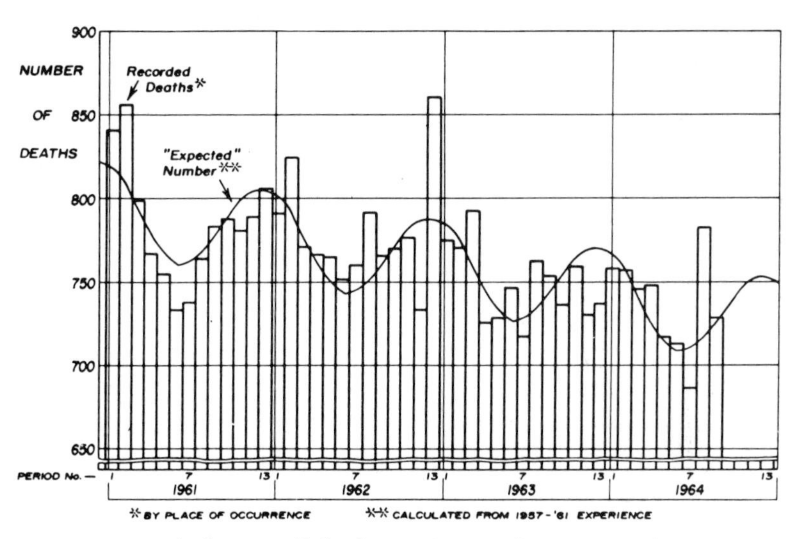


*Figure 9. Graph showing all deaths in infants under one year of age in 108 cities in the United States. They are increased in the winter months. The highest bars probably represent epidemics of acute respiratory disease. From the United States Public Health Service.*

hypothesis at this time would tend to suggest that the baby's first experience with respiratory viruses may be overwhelming and that a "cold of the lungs" is sufficient to interfere with vital and essential ventilation, leading to sharply reduced supplies of oxygen and sudden unexpected death.

# 13 "Strep" Throats and Other Bacterial Infections

The main concern in this chapter will be with the streptococcus as a relatively common cause of throat infections related to bacteria. We are not concerned with the streptococcus as a cause of common colds, but primarily because it must be differentiated from other infections which may simulate a cold. Certain adenovirus infections, influenza, and infectious mononucleosis may be impossible to separate from streptococcal infections. The rare cases of diphtheria may occasionally be confused and should also be considered in the differential diagnosis.

Most of the evidence supports the idea that the pneumococcus, staphylococcus, influenza bacillus, and meningococcus are complicating secondary infections preceded by or working together with a viral infection. The main symptoms may relate to the secondary bacterial invader, particularly when toxic signs and other complications dominate the symptoms. Swollen glands in the neck, earache, and sometimes severe croup and bronchitis may be related to the secondary germs. Where this fact has become clear, antibiotics have been employed commonly in the treatment of these complications. It soon became evident, however, that swollen glands in the neck and ear infections, as well as pneumonia, might be caused by the primary virus infection, and antibiotics were often found ineffective in treatment. Great clinical skill and judgment are often required to determine the role of bacteria in such apparent complications of primary infection. Although swollen glands and ear infections may be due to viruses, they do represent extension of diseases from the throat and often in themselves provide an indication for the use of antibiotics or antibacterial drugs.

There are several large groups of streptococci, but the commonest one to infect human beings is designated as group A. Under group A there are nearly 50 subtypes, and these are quite distinctive, separating these organisms one from another. After having survived a natural infection from one of the types of streptococcus, the victim is rendered immune; evidence of a return infection by the same type in the same individual is rare indeed.

"Strep" throats are characterized by sudden onset, with extreme soreness, fever, and certain constitutional symptoms such as headache and weakness. The throat appears bright red, as does the skin rash, when present. No doubt the term "scarlet fever" has been derived from this. Many patients with a "strep throat" infection have a greyish white membrane on the tonsils or throat. The membrane may appear after from 24 to 36 hours, but when the patient is seen early it may *not* be evident. Inflammation in the throat is intense and often leads to mild bleeding.

The streptococcus is capable of producing many different illnesses in addition to throat infection and enlarged glands in the neck. It may cause skin infections such as impetigo or erysipelas. Pneumonia, pleurisy (empyema), meningitis, and mastoiditis are known to be caused by this organism. Rarer diseases such as osteomyelitis, heart infections, and vaginitis may be caused by "strep." Dr. Burtis B. Breese, a long-time student of streptococcal diseases, states that the vast majority are infections of the throat and that approximately 10 per cent of these are scarlet fever. He points out that the late consequences of these infections, rheumatic heart disease and inflammation of the kidneys (nephritis), occur in a small percentage of patients; and it is for this reason that streptococcal infections are so important. If treated early and adequately, these complications can largely be prevented. This places great responsibility on the physician to make an accurate diagnosis of sore throats early, in order to prevent serious complications.

Certain additional tests are extremely important in arriving at an accurate diagnosis. Dr. Breese emphasizes the value of a high white blood cell count, usually 15,000 or more. Counts are rarely under this in a true streptococcal infection. The classic symptoms of the common cold such as coryza, cough, and hoarseness are not commonly associated with streptococcal infections and may be most helpful in separating one from another. Hoarseness as a symptom is most commonly associated with nonbacterial infections of the throat. In "strep" infections, mothers will often describe the child's voice as "thick" rather than "hoarse."

In infancy and in the preschool child streptococcal infections tend to be less dramatic than in older children and young adults. The illness is frequently accompanied by low grade fever with loss of appetite and a heavy discharge from the nose. Between six months and three years a low grade illness may persist for many weeks, with mild inflammation of the throat and a nasal discharge that is often profuse.

Scarlet fever is more common in the age group from three to ten years, and acute tonsillitis or sore throat is the most significant finding. The rash of scarlet fever appears first on the body, often in the folds of the arm, and rarely involves the face—where a flush is common, with paleness about the mouth. The rash feels bumpy, and this feature may appear even before redness. The rash may also appear in the mouth, and the tongue presents a typical strawberry appearance.

A wide range of symptoms and signs may be caused by the streptococcus, and the spectrum is always important to keep in mind. In family studies carried out in Cleveland, Ohio, over the past ten years, the streptococcus accounted for about 2½ per cent of all respiratory illnesses. It is important to remember that many other nonstreptococcal infections may cause white spots on the tonsils, and certainly acute sore throat and enlarged glands in the neck are much more commonly caused by other infectious agents. The mere culturing of the germ does not establish the infection as being due to streptococcus, but a sharp rise in antibodies in the blood is most convincing evidence. In certain forms of nonstreptococcal tonsillitis, when the streptococcal organism is found by culture, as many as half of the cases fail to show a rise in antibodies or evidence that the infection is actually due to the streptococcus. Cultures, on the other hand, are extremely helpful; when the growth is luxuriant, the evidence warrants a positive clinical diagnosis. When a heavy growth occurs, associated with typical symptoms, little doubt should remain as to the indications for treatment. There are several important reasons for treating the patient: (1) to ameliorate the symptoms, (2) to prevent complications, (3) to eradicate the organism, and (4) to prevent its spread to other individuals.

A few strains of streptococcus have been reported to be resistant to the sulfa drugs, but most of them are highly sensitive to penicillin, which still remains the drug of choice for the treatment of streptococcal infections. A minimum of ten days of treatment is important in order to prevent complications and to eliminate the organism.

Although extremely rare, diphtheria must be kept in mind when infections occur in the tonsils and throat. There is real danger of becoming complacent about diphtheria, which may occur in the incompletely immunized individual or when immunity is allowed to reach a low level. The membrane in the throat in diphtheria is often more extensive than in nonbacterial or streptococcal sore throat. The discharge may be bloody, and the odor is offensive. Swelling in the neck occurs, associated with difficulty in swallowing and noisy breathing, often with complete loss of voice. Treatment consists of early diagnosis and the use of antitoxin plus penicillin, which should be administered in full therapeutic doses for at least ten days.

Whooping cough is an important disease and causes more deaths in the first year of life than measles, scarlet fever, diphtheria, and poliomyelitis combined. In the early stages of this disease, there is no way to differentiate the cough from one caused by many other agents. Early diagnosis is important in order to begin treatment early and thus minimize the severity and deaths from these infections. A high white blood cell count with predominant lymph cells may be very helpful in diagnosis, but methods using cultures should also be employed. Wide-spectrum antibiotics are helpful, particularly when begun early in the course of illness. Effective prevention is the ultimate key to the eradication of whooping cough.

In summary, the streptococcus is one of the few bacteria which may apparently *initiate* a throat infection. Most organisms found in the nose and throat cause infection on top of a viral illness such as measles or influenza. Scarlet fever represents about one tenth of throat infections due to streptococcus. Tonsillitis caused by streptococcus may simulate flu, adenovirus, infectious mononucleosis, diphtheria, and other illnesses. Infection by the streptococcus may occur with no symptoms or very mild symptoms. Whooping cough may simulate a hard cold with little or no fever.

# 14 Q Fever and "Parrot Fever" or Psittacosis

Q fever, an acute illness with fever, although rare compared with other diseases, must be considered in any influenzalike or common cold illness. Cough occurs in a certain percentage of these patients, but fever and general aching with severe headache are the commonest symptoms. An X ray of the chest may reveal unsuspected shadows. The germ that causes Q fever is a rickettsial organism closely related to viruses. It may be found by inoculating the blood of individuals into certain susceptible animals.

The incubation period may be long, from 14 to 26 days with an average of 19, followed by headache and fever with loss of appetite. Mild dry cough develops in most cases, and many complain of pain in the chest. Even mildly ill patients may show evidence of a spot of pneumonia on the X-ray film of the chest. There are very few characteristic findings in this disease, as it may simulate many influenzalike illnesses.

The epidemiological features are of interest, as the disease is often associated with workers in slaughterhouses. It is transmitted in nature by ticks; slaughterhouse workers undoubtedly contract the disease by inhaling dust from hides that have been contaminated. An epidemic was reported from a hair processing plant in Philadelphia, Pennsylvania, which involved 30 employees. The disease was an acute illness, which was referred to as the flu or grippe. When the blood of many of the employees was studied, it was found that 67 individuals had positive tests for Q fever. The organism that causes Q fever *does* respond to wide-spectrum antibiotics, and they should always be employed in the treatment of this disease.

"Parrot fever" was first recognized in the Psittacine birds as an acute infectious disease known to involve many different species of birds, which may transfer the illness to human beings at all ages. In general the infection is mild or inapparent but occasionally can produce a severe illness with a high mortality. The causative agent is no longer considered to be a virus, but it is closely related. It is possible that transmission may occur from one sick individual to another, although most infections are probably acquired from handling birds. The disease is constantly present in parakeet aviaries as well as in pigeon and duck breeding establishments. Pigeons, ducks, and chickens may harbor the germ, and the highest incidence of infection is recorded in women who are bird fanciers and engage in breeding of birds. Transmission, however, occurs by air, from handling of sick or dead birds, or by the excreta from birds that may be harboring a hidden infection.

An epidemic in Louisiana caused eight deaths and many proved illnesses among nursing attendants. More recently state and federal control measures have resulted in a marked decrease in the spread of infection. The disease is now almost eliminated in many states.

The history of contact with sick birds is often helpful, but is not necessary to make the diagnosis. Sore throat, headache, and chills are early symptoms of parrot fever. A cough may develop which persists for several weeks. Parrot fever may occur at all ages, but it is relatively rare in children, probably due to less intimate exposure. Antibiotics should be used in the treatment of psittacosis, as they may be life-saving in this serious disease. The sulfa drugs as well as penicillin have been reported to be beneficial in treatment. The dosage should be determined by the severity of the illness and the recommendation of the physician in charge.

Strict isolation of patients with parrot fever is highly recommended because the agent may be present up to the third week of illness. It is important to dispose of all excretions, and a strenuous search should be made for the source of infection. Healthy birds may harbor the agent, and birds that appear well are frequently of more importance than visibly sick birds.

The writer was once asked to testify in defense of a father and mother who were accused of killing their three-month-old-baby, found dead in his crib. The findings at the time of the post-mortem examination consisted of an enlarged spleen (twice normal size) and pneumonia in small areas of the lung. Neither of these findings was considered very significant until it turned out on careful questioning that a pair of parakeets had been purchased about three weeks prior to the death of the baby. One of the birds was found dead in the cage the same day the baby died, and the other bird died a week later. When the store from which they were purchased was investigated, it had closed with no sign of the fly-by-night salesman or owner.

A careful review of the autopsy findings revealed the characteristic changes compatible with those found in patients with parrot fever. The brain of the baby showed some congestion in addition to the large spleen and virus-like pneumonia. The young couple was acquitted by the jury.

# 15 Fungal Infections and Tuberculosis

Acute respiratory diseases or common colds may often be simulated by fungal infections of the respiratory passages. There are two important diseases caused by fungi in the United States, both of which may be a mild influenzalike illness followed by rapid recovery. Skin tests similar to the tuberculin test have established the fact that these agents produce inapparent illness in a large percentage of infected individuals. The first disease to be discussed is "San Joaquin Valley fever," known as *coccidioidomycosis* and spoken of commonly by the medical profession as "cocci." The second fungal disease is *histoplasmosis;* the highest incidence of infection by the latter fungus is concentrated in the rainy mid-central United States around the junction of the Ohio and Mississippi rivers. The peak incidence of "cocci" occurs in the southwestern United States, and, in sharp contrast to histoplasmosis, it thrives in extremely dry areas. The endemic centers for these two diseases are separated by more than 2,000 miles, but rapid shifts in population and travel habits have resulted in a wide dispersion of both of these diseases, which have now been recognized throughout the United States. They both may invade the respiratory passages and produce mild illness in man. They also, on rare occasions, can produce severe and overwhelming infection, the nature of which will be described briefly in the following paragraphs dealing with each disease.

The fungus that causes "Valley fever" or "cocci" thrives in the soil and when disturbed may be carried by winds for long distances. New housing developments have produced epidemics in the area of digging; the disease is recognized to be common among archeologists, who also like to dig. The onset of illness occurs one to three weeks following exposure to contaminated dust. The striking symptoms are low grade fever and cough. The infection has been reported to be so mild that many individuals escape any outward signs of illness. The disease, however, can be detected by the skin sensitivity test which becomes positive a few weeks after infection. It has been estimated that 30 to 40 per cent of exposed patients who become infected develop an illness, which they call "desert fever," or a "cold," or "the grippe."

In addition to the fever and cough, which are the first symptoms, the more severely ill develop chest pain, and occasionally the patient will spit up blood following an attack of coughing. X-ray studies of the chest reveal shadows, and sometimes fluid is seen surrounding the lung. The infection may become progressive and spread throughout the body, including the brain and its coverings. The systemic form of the disease occurs in approximately one-quarter of one per cent of Caucasians. The incidence in Negroes may be 10 to 30 times as high. At one time in the early stages of our knowledge regarding these two diseases, both were considered highly fatal. In 1938 it was discovered that "cocci" can be a very mild infection. At the far end of the spectrum, when the fungus gets into the blood, nearly every organ in the body may be involved, including the brain.

The writer has observed this disease in a seven-month-old infant who lived in an area near the ocean considered to be quite free of this infection. A careful history revealed that the child was taken through the San Joaquin Valley in an automobile on *one* occasion. A sore on the baby's lip was apparently the earliest sign, and it was not until swelling of the fingers occurred as a result of infection in the bones that the patient was taken to the family doctor. X-ray studies revealed that several bones of the body were involved with destructive changes. The baby's liver and spleen were enlarged. In spite of all of these severe changes, he was quite free of fever, eating well, and gaining weight. He continued to improve without any special treatment and after three years is now considered to be quite well.

Most of the common antibiotics have failed to show any beneficial effect in the severe form of this disease. Recently amphotericin B has been found to have antifungal properties and has been used with real benefit in many patients with the severe forms of "Valley fever."

The second fungus disease, histoplasmosis, is widespread in the United States. By means of the skin test, histoplasmosis has been found to occur with a high rate of frequency in densely populated areas. Histoplasmosis may mimic many other diseases, and in its milder forms it cannot be separated from common maladies such as influenza and unexplained fever until additional tests are performed. The widespread use of the tuberculin test and chest X rays revealed that many patients had evidence of spots of calcium in the lung with a negative test to tuberculin. Many of these patients were found to have a positive test to histoplasmin, and again, as in "cocci" and tuberculosis, it was learned that this disease occurs in mild or inapparent forms in the majority of persons infected. The classic findings are those of fever, slight cough, and chest pain. The symptoms are closely related to those just described for coccidioidomycosis. In epidemics, the illness is characterized by a wide spectrum varying from inapparent and very mild illness to extremely severe disease. Those who are heavily exposed and receive a large dose may suffer from very severe forms of the disease, which are most common in the very young.

The chronic form of histoplasmosis is recognized as similar to tuberculosis and characterized by ups and downs with intermittent influenzalike illnesses.

This fungus is found in the soil and may be transmitted directly to man and animals. It appears to thrive in shady, damp areas, particularly in enclosures such as chicken coops, pigeon roosts, and storm cellars. No treatment is indicated for the milder forms of this disease, and the outlook for recovery is very favorable in the great majority; exceptions, of course, are the overwhelming severe forms and occasionally the chronic forms of disease, where treatment with antifungal drugs is indicated.

■

The following brief discussion of one of the world's most important diseases will be limited to the *primary* forms of infection caused by the tubercle bacillus. Many of these illnesses simulate respiratory disease and pass for a mild, moderate, or sometimes severe cold lasting varying periods of time. If it were not for the tuberculin test, one of the finest of all tests in medicine, we might be quite unaware of the fact that this serious disease occurs in inapparent and mild forms. A positive skin test indicates that the individual has been infected and has become sensitive to the protein of the tubercle bacillus. The tuberculin test is highly efficient and when properly applied *in the skin,* it is by far the most effective means available to separate persons who have been infected from those who have not. Repeated testing is the best means of detecting early tuberculosis; certain individuals who have been infected mildly and develop a positive reaction may change back to a negative test in surprisingly high numbers. It was once thought that if the tuberculin test is positive, it remained so for the rest of one's life, but this is now known not to be the case.

Because of the tuberculin test, primary tuberculosis is probably the *first* disease in which a wide clinical spectrum was recognized and established. It is apparent that many individuals acquire their first infection without any knowledge of illness or have a vague ill-defined illness similar to a cold, with a cough and low grade fever. If a chest X ray is taken, the findings are often startling when compared to the patient's symptoms. These early first infections in childhood tend to heal up completely in well-nourished individuals. In countries of the world where malnutrition is widespread, the incidence of tuberculosis is very high.

Dr. Johannes Holm, Executive Director of the International Union against Tuberculosis, expresses great concern for the complacency toward this "serious and even dangerous" situation. He states that the public is misinformed about the actual tuberculosis problem in being told that it no longer exists. Dr. M. G. Candau, Director General of the World Health Organization, states that "at least 15,-000,000 people suffer from infectious tuberculosis in the world today and the disease still claims more than 3,000,-000 lives annually." It is true that the decline in tuberculosis deaths has been spectacular in many of our highly developed countries, but the number of tuberculosis sufferers has not declined as rapidly as the deaths. It is conservatively estimated that between 2 and 3 million new cases still occur each year.

In some less developed areas of the world 70 per cent of children may be infected before they reach the age of 14. In Latin America there are 600,000 known cases of active tuberculosis and probably 1,800,000 undeclared. The World Health Committee on Tuberculosis reports that the disease could not be considered to be eliminated as a public health problem unless the number of children who become infected before the age of 14 fell below one per cent. They state further that not a single country in the world today satisfies this condition—yet for the first time in the history of man we possess effective weapons to fight tuberculosis.

Dr. James E. Perkins of the National Tuberculosis Association stated in April 1964: "As tuberculosis knows no geographic or racial boundaries, it is everyone's problem and will continue to be until the disease is eliminated—whether country by country or continent by continent. But even in a country like the United States where the death rate is down, more than 53,000 new cases are reported a year. The battle is far from won and, until it is, *there can be no truce for tuberculosis.*"

# 16 Allergic Diseases: Hay Fever and Asthma

In a discussion of allergy and colds, a clear definition of terms becomes important. Dr. John H. Dingle in his presidential address before the American Association of Immunologists pointed out that although a tremendous number of papers representing extensive observations and investigations exist in the world literature, it is curious that the common cold remains so elusive and difficult to define. He states that "a sharp definition of the common cold is not possible" and that we should probably leave the definition to the patient, who simply speaks of a "head cold" or a "chest cold."

"Coryza" is a running nose, and the term "rhinorrhea" also indicates a thin nasal discharge frequently referred to as a cold. Allergic rhinitis might easily be confused with infectious rhinitis. Thus several factors, such as allergic responses in the nose, viral infections in the nose, and bacterial and even psychosomatic disturbances may produce rhinorrhea. Many known agents numbering more than a hundred manifest themselves with symptoms and signs of what people call a "cold." Allergic rhinitis includes both hay fever and allergic disorders which are common during the pollination season, the latter tending to occur in the warmest months of the year. Allergic rhinitis may not be seasonal and is commonly diagnosed as a cold. House dust, occupational dust, molds, and animal danders, including feathers and wool in garments and blankets, make up some of the common inhalants that cause trouble. Certain foods and drugs may precipitate symptoms and occasionally sensitivity to bacteria will cause allergic rhinitis. A combination of causes leads to confusion. It is possible that an allergic reaction may predispose to bacterial infection, which in turn may respond to antibiotics. Primary allergic congestion may respond to antiallergic drugs, such as antihistamines. They are of little or no avail in the treatment of virus colds.

Uncomplicated allergic rhinitis causes less redness of the nasal membranes than infections. Symptoms of allergic disease are often associated with itching in the nose. Chronic unproductive cough may result from the same sensory disturbances in the throat and bronchial tubes. The frequently recurring or "continuous cold" of childhood is nearly always due to allergic nasal mucous membranes. A history in the family of allergic conditions is helpful, but true allergic disease may be unknown, and terms such as chronic sinusitis and bronchitis may be prominent. An increased number of cells, called *eosinophils,* in the secretions of the nose may be helpful in differentiating these "head cold" problems. Chronic rhinitis in infants may be directly related to allergy to cow's milk. Associated sinusitis and bronchitis with chronic cough often accompany an allergic condition.

When chronic disease is present in the nose and sinuses, a dual attack on allergy and infection may be important to consider. It is clear that diagnosis and management often go hand in hand, as elimination of house dust, pollens, and so forth may play a prominent part in the relief of the patient's symptoms. A combination of antibiotics and allergic management will sometimes bring good results. The first step should include antiallergic measures, which by themselves may bring prompt relief. A reduction in pollen sensitivity usually consists of injecting gradually increasing doses of an extract of the pollens to which the patient is allergic. This method, combined with antihistamine treatment, may give marked relief to the victim of seasonal hay fever.

In summary, bronchial asthma is characterized by cough and wheezing caused by swelling of the lining membranes of the bronchi. The guilty offenders may be pollens or inhalants, foods, drugs, and many other substances. Acute respiratory infections often bring on an asthmatic attack or make it worse. The two seem to go together in the fall and winter seasons. Sudden changes in temperature, exertion, or emotional disturbances likewise play a significant role in the severity of asthma. The problem is a complex one with no clear solution.

# 17 Serious Complications and After-effects of Colds

It is important to remind ourselves once again of some basic concepts—namely, the wide clinical spectrum of illness and the significance of naming diseases when possible according to their causes. Acute respiratory diseases, known to be caused by many different viruses, are generally mild, self-limited illnesses. In many instances the majority of these infections may be entirely inapparent, as previously emphasized for polio, influenza, primary tuberculosis, and several others. The concern in this chapter is with the *rare,* far end of the spectrum, the very serious illnesses that may result in death or damaging aftereffects. Brain fever, inflammation of the heart, and pneumonia (sometimes occurring together) are the commonest serious complications.

Meningoencephalitis, which implies inflammation of the brain and its coverings, occurs rarely in association with nearly all of the diseases discussed in this book. A closer look at common measles will serve to point up the importance of the rare occurrence of measles encephalitis, the most serious manifestation of this common world-wide disease. Recent estimates have indicated that the incidence of encephalitis in the United States is 1 to 1.5 per 1,000 reported cases of measles. In virgin areas like Greenland, the rate has been recorded at 6 per 1,000. No consistent relationship between the *severity* of measles and involvement of the nervous system is apparent. Encephalitis may occur in association with the milder forms of measles even after gamma globulin has been given. When the eruption appears many patients become drowsy and even slightly stuporous but fail to develop any further neurologic symptoms.

The onset of encephalitis is commonly from two to five days after the appearance of rash, but in a number of reported cases encephalitis has actually preceded the rash by one to five days. When the disease begins, irritability and even convulsions may usher in the ominous attack of encephalitis. Convulsions may be followed by coma or the gradual progression into a stupor, following the onset of headache, vomiting, and restlessness. These signs are usually accompanied by high fever with stiffness of the neck and signs of tremor or muscle twitching. Except for the most severe cases, these features tend to disappear in a few days, but stupor may rarely persist for weeks. The patient may exhibit emotional instability by becoming easily excited and upset. Certain speech defects, such as slurring of words or complete loss of voice, are not uncommon. Blindness or drooping of the eyelid occurs rarely. Difficulties with the bladder and bowel may be evident, with weakness of the legs.

The recovery rate from measles encephalitis is variable and tends to be less favorable in the very young, who may have experienced convulsions and coma. Mental impairment is a most serious aftereffect, and it may be associated with behavior disturbances. Brain wave tests or electroencephalograms show a characteristic pattern in these children, which may clear up but also may persist and be accompanied by a convulsive disorder. It is not uncommon for complications to be associated with measles encephalitis; acute blindness has been recorded in several patients.

No specific treatment has been found effective in measles encephalitis. In New York City, 159 cases with this serious form of measles, all under the age of 15 years, were observed closely over a 5½-year period. Fifty-one had received adequate amounts of gamma globulin, and 108 had not. Approximately a quarter of these cases died or had permanent aftereffects. The percentage was the same in both groups.

The actual direct cause of measles encephalitis has not been determined, and the disease has usually been classified as postinfectious encephalitis. This label implies that the virus of measles does not cause this complication but that it is an aftereffect possibly related to an "allergic" type of response. This idea has no real basis in fact as the cause of measles encephalitis. Many other socalled postinfectious encephalitides, including those following vaccination for smallpox, mumps, and chicken pox, have been shown to be due to the virus. The changes in the brain in all of these instances may be quite similar. They are characterized by a loss of myelin (the covering of the nerves), which disappears in certain areas of the brain.

Encephalitis has been reported in association with nearly all of the common contagious diseases, and when it occurs it has many of the features just reviewed in the instance of common measles. In the chapter concerned with infectious mononucleosis, infectious lymphocytosis, and lymphocytic choriomeningitis brief mention was made of the association of encephalitis with all three. It has been stated that the incidence of involvement of the nervous system in infectious mononucleosis may occur in 1 to 2 per cent of the proved cases. The signs of nervous involvement begin 10 to 14 days after the onset of illness and may be very severe with mental confusion, convulsions, and coma. In the case of lymphocytic choriomeningitis, one report tells of the occurrence of this illness in the newborn baby following an illness in the mother 12 days prior to delivery. Six days after birth the baby became ill, and six days later he died. The virus was isolated from the baby's spinal fluid and from the brain at post-mortem examination. The virus was also isolated from house mice caught in the home.

The important association of encephalitis is found in many of the 60 or more enteroviruses including poliomyelitis, Coxsackie, and echovirus infections. It was emphasized earlier in Chapter IX that all of these agents may on occasion be associated with summer colds and flulike illnesses and occasionally with rash illnesses most commonly seen in the summer months. Muscle weakness and paralysis as well as other neurological signs have been observed in certain of the Coxsackie and echovirus infections, and in some cases aftereffects have persisted. The onset of nervous symptoms may be abrupt or gradual, featured by headache, fever, and stiff neck. Abdominal pain may be common. The isolation of poliovirus from the spinal fluid has occurred only rarely, but poliovirus has been found with ease in the case of the Coxsackie B viruses and several of the A types, as well as echoviruses.

Involvement of the heart with inflammation is a very important finding in poliomyelitis occurring in as many as a fifth of the hospitalized cases. Carditis has been a most serious complication of Coxsackie B infections, particularly in newborn infants, in whom it is a highly fatal disease. Several epidemics of Coxsackie B in infants have been reported. The first of these was observed in Johannesburg in 1952 and involved ten babies, six of whom died after a feverish disease with heart failure. The Coxsackie virus was isolated from several of these patients. Dr. van Creveld observed four cases of acute carditis in newborns in association with an epidemic of "summer grippe" in adults in Amsterdam in 1955. This epidemic was proved to be related to Coxsackie B virus. He reports that some of the mothers of these babies showed symptoms of influenza.

In one study, 25 infants infected with Coxsackie B virus were reported, with a mortality of 76 per cent, indicating the violent nature of this disorder. A report from England of carditis with croup caused by Coxsackie virus B tells of four cases due to this virus in children aged 4 to 19 months. These cases occurred during a period when Coxsackie virus infections were prevalent in the general population. Two of the cases had acute heart inflammation, one had inflammation of the heart and croup, and the fourth had croup only. All of these patients, being in the older (older than newborns) age group, recovered from their disease. The fact that one infant had *only* croup from this virus infection is of real interest and emphasizes again the "clinical spectrum" of illness.

As a part of the wide spectrum, pneumonia may occur in association with nearly all viral infections and may be due to the virus itself or a combination of virus and bacteria. Pneumonia as a complication of an otherwise mild illness probably accounts for the majority mortality that may be associated with any of these infections. Several of these have been discussed in more detail in Chapter X, concerned with virus pneumonias.

Very little is known of the incidence of inapparent encephalitis associated with the more severe manifestations of common virus infections. Brain wave studies in uncomplicated measles and poliomyelitis have shown a surprisingly high incidence (nearly 50 per cent) of abnormal findings, which fortunately return to normal in a matter of days or weeks. Months later they are most difficult to correlate for certain with the original illness. Probably the best evidence for the late aftereffects is established in the instance of common measles.

The incidence of convulsive disorders in children is much higher in patients who have recovered from encephalitis usually of unknown cause. Now that recent advances have made it possible to identify many of these milder illnesses, the correlation of neurological disturbances may be possible. In the case of uncomplicated mumps and chicken pox, spinal fluid studies have shown that children with *no* neurologic signs may have abnormal changes in their spinal fluid. This is clear evidence of very mild or inapparent encephalitis. Fortunately, immediate or prompt recovery takes place; but the aftereffects, which may appear months or years later, are the unfortunate side of the problem. The importance of these relationships cannot be overemphasized when the prevalence of mentally handicapping conditions is recognized. The future holds promise that our understanding of many of these distressing conditions will increase as a result of the rapid progress being made in our knowledge of the basic causes of the commonest diseases of man.

# 18 The Management of the Child's First Cold

Colds are the most common of all illnesses, and fortunately most of them are mild. They will even seem to be unimportant, but they are a very definite and important part of growing up. Most of them will make the child resistant or protect him from having the same "virus cold" a second or third time. Like regular measles, he will be protected from a second attack. The problem is that so many different viruses (over 100) may cause colds that it becomes a vital part of life to have these experiences with many different colds.

Almost all colds are a mild form of a virus infection, but they can occasionally be serious and involve the lungs or other organs of the body. When this happens the symptoms and signs are usually obvious, if we are aware that they can occur. The fever will be higher than with an ordinary cold. This is not a bad sign and may even be helpful in the process of getting well. When we have a virus infection, the body's cell makes a substance called "interferon." It was so named because it interferes with the growth and spread of viruses and so is a most important way the body has of recovering from the virus attack. Interferon works best to help us recover in the presence of some fever, so we now believe that we should not rush to give aspirin for every little bout of fever, but use our judgment and give it only when the fever seems to interfere with rest. In most instances, moderately high fevers are not too disturbing to the baby. High fevers require the attention of your doctor.

When should the doctor be called? Almost *anytime* if you are worried about the baby. The doctor will talk about the symptoms and then decide whether it is necessary to make a more complete examination. It is often helpful to take the baby's temperature before calling the doctor. He will want to know if the baby has been exposed to someone with an illness, or if others in the family are ill. Coughs, vomiting, or loose bowel movements are important symptoms, too. He will ask if the baby is taking liquids and how much.

Certainly it is not necessary to call the doctor every time the baby seems to have a cold. Sneezing, running nose, and a little cough are usually not serious symptoms; when fever, restlessness, and a hard cough appear, it is wise to inform the doctor and ask his advice. He probably will want to see the baby before prescribing medicine. Do not be disturbed if he chooses not to give medicine, as there is no specific drug for most colds. He may give you advice for feeding and ways to promote rest. He will tell you what to watch for and ask you to keep him informed of new symptoms.

After most colds the child will develop antibodies, and these will be helpful to protect him from another attack, so all is not in vain. When symptoms seem to recur before the cold has gone away, it may be a new virus rather than a relapse or further invasion by the previous one. On the other hand, it may also be a secondary complication or a germ, like a bacterium, which often makes us ill by working together with the viruses that cause colds. Bacteria may get into the lungs to cause bronchitis or pneumonia, or they may get into the inner ear to cause what is called *otitis media*. Sometimes the glands in the neck become inflamed following hard colds and throat infections. Tonsillitis may be a part of the virus infection, or it may be caused by bacteria such as the streptococcus (Chapter XIII). Hoarseness is usually an early symptom of a virus infection and rarely occurs with the bacterial forms, when a "thick" voice is more common.

Measles is one of the most serious virus infections; it causes all the symptoms of a cold (cough, coryza, and conjunctivitis) and then is accompanied by a blotchy rash in nearly all instances. A safe and very effective vaccine is available and should be given to everyone who has not had regular measles. If there is any reason not to give the vaccine, your doctor will tell you. The measles virus may cause pneumonia by itself or invite bacteria to attack. The most serious illness associated with measles is the rare involvement of the brain which occurs in about one case per thousand. This may not sound very common to you, but if it affects *your* child it is common enough. With about 4,000,000 cases of measles a year in the United States, this means 4,000 children will have encephalitis, and many of those who survive will have brain damage for life. Do not wait to have the child vaccinated!

Everyone seems willing to give advice about the best way to treat your cold. Radio and television promote their remedies in various forms many times a day. Millions of dollars are spent to get relief or to find a cure. The best treatment is very inexpensive: rest! Most physicians, I think, will agree that you cannot "run off" or "work off" a cold; no special diet has proved to be beneficial, but perhaps eating as desired, with emphasis on plenty of liquids, is sensible. Aspirin should be avoided unless indicated or prescribed by your doctor, as fever may actually be part of the body's defense. Interferon, as explained previously, is more effective in the presence of fever. Citrus fruits such as orange juice have many proponents. It certainly is not harmful, but it also has not been proved to have any special curative effect for colds. As Thomas Phaire said in 1553, "The beste and moste sure help in this case is not to meddle with anye kynde of medicines, but to let nature worke her operacio."

Are colds just nuisance diseases anyway? The facts are quite the contrary. Many viruses such as the influenzas may cause serious infections and death. In 1957, 78,000 deaths were attributed to Asian flu. More babies are found dead in their cribs during epidemics of respiratory disease. Pneumonia nearly always begins as a mild illness often referred to as a cold. Meningitis may and often does start as a cold. The viruses which rarely cause inflammation of the heart (carditis) and brain (encephalitis) may be colds at one stage of the infection; so even though most colds are mild illnesses, they are important and should be respected. Rest accomplishes two things—it not only aids our recovery but also keeps us from spreading our germs to others outside the family. Do not hesitate to share your concern with your doctor; he is also concerned!

The author frequently advocates "postural drainage" to treat cough and prevent infections in the nose and throat from getting into the lungs. With a firm mattress under the baby, he is often happiest when on his stomach and face down. Usually the head is turned to one side or the other. When a baby is on his back, the dangers of choking on mucus or food is much greater, and when vomiting he should be turned over at once. Babies can be taught to sleep in this position from early in life, as shown in the accompanying picture (Figure 10).

What can be done to protect other members of the family? Older children frequently bring the colds home from school. The incidence of colds is higher for the baby who has older brothers and sisters. The problem is that children or any of us may have cold viruses and not have symptoms, or we may be spreading the germs a few days before the start of a cold. These facts make it almost impossible to prevent infection within the family, but intimate contact and kissing should be avoided. Remember, colds are very contagious, particularly for those who have not had that particular cold before. The wearing of a mask

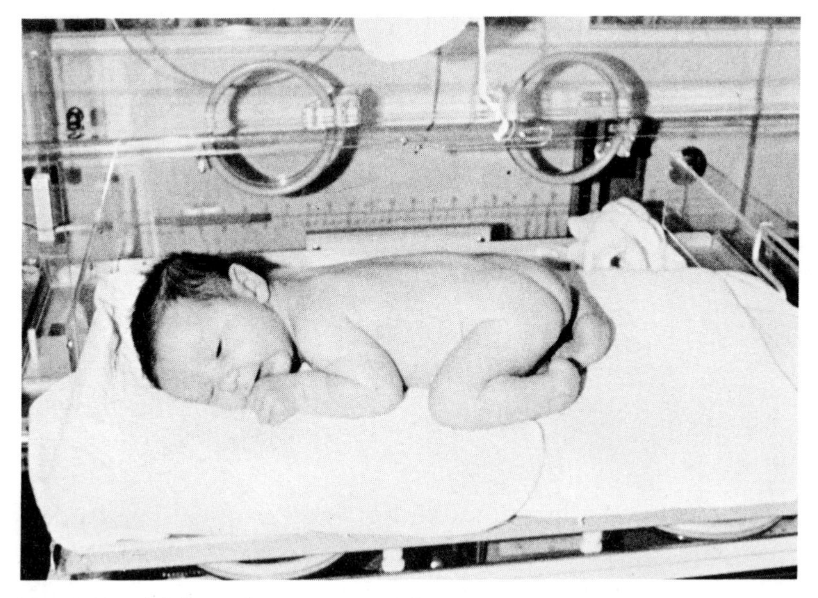

*Figure 10. A baby in the prone or face-down position.*

over the nose and mouth does little good and is most uncomfortable for the wearer. It is, however, a warning to others to stay away.

# 19 The Outlook for the Ultimate Control and Effective Treatment of Colds

Most authorities are willing to express optimism regarding the control of acute respiratory diseases. At the same time they express real concern and caution regarding any *quick* solutions to these highly complex problems. Several vaccines have been developed in the past few years, and along with this progress many difficulties have arisen. At the present time, safe and effective vaccines would appear to be the most logical approach. Advances in virology, particularly the adaptation to tissue culture, have come about more rapidly than the acquisition of information regarding the effects of vaccines on the body.

Years of research in the fields of influenza and poliomyelitis have provided a great deal of basic epidemiological and clinical knowledge, which is essential to the development of an effective control program. This kind of information is necessary for the newly recognized viruses before effective controls can be established. One of the first steps, aside from isolating viruses from sick individuals, is to determine the natural history and relative importance of each of the viruses implicated. An effective program will require broad, comprehensive, and controlled studies in various populations during all seasons and continuing for several years.

The director of a large institute for therapeutic research summarizes the problem of future vaccines with this statement: "There are at present sufficient data and adequate technology to permit and to justify a concerted effort toward the development of vaccines which give promise of controlling a sizeable portion of the total respiratory disease spectrum." He, too, adds a word of caution by stating that "the problem of control of respiratory disease by vaccination is complex and much more lies ahead than behind. . . . the conquest of respiratory illness seems a trivial task compared with the conquest of space."

Vaccines for smallpox and rabies have been available for many years. The vaccinia virus, closely related to the smallpox virus, has eradicated the disease from many parts of the world. Yet today the World Health Organization reports thousands of cases annually occurring in underdeveloped countries. Yellow fever and polio vaccines have been developed with great success in more recent times. Measles prevention with live weakened forms of the virus is highly effective and safe. The vaccine in its present form is expensive and as yet is not employed widely in the world. Influenza and adenovirus are being developed and improved by constant research. The most recent vaccines are discussed in detail in Chapters IV and VI, which deal with these diseases.

The problem of the direct treatment of acute viral respiratory illness has been a most discouraging one compared to the dramatic effects of antibiotics against bacteria and spirochetes (parasites that cause syphilis). Dr. Robert R. Wagner writes that "contrary to popular opinion it is not difficult to inhibit virus multiplication. The problem, of course, rests on injuring the cell which has already been invaded by the virus by the time the disease is evident." Dr. Wagner focuses attention on the virus-infected cell rather than on the virus. In order to do so it is important to understand the chemical composition and the way viruses act and effect the cell.

Antibodies appear to prevent the penetration of virus into the cell; the effectiveness of antibodies is largely limited to prevention. They probably do not alter the course of acute viral disease largely because the response is too late, and it is recognized that certain infections progress even in the presence of large amounts of circulating antibodies.

Interferon was discussed briefly in Chapter 1 and is mentioned again merely to point out that it is a substance produced by body cells infected with many different viruses. It has no particular *specificity* for the type of virus that initiated its production. It reacts with the cell and interferes with virus multiplication. Interferon appears to be much more active in tissue culture than in the living body. This is probably simply a matter of the dose required to treat an infection. Hopefully this problem may be solved if methods can be devised for obtaining more potent preparations.

Researchers at the Rockefeller Institute in New York, discovered that strange enzymes were produced by the infected cells. They found that a chemical called HBB could stop or interfere with the growth of viruses. *Guanidine* and HBB were especially effective against the large group of picornaviruses; these are polio, Coxsackie, echo, and rhinoviruses in particular. They work against the enzymes and thus prevent the viruses from growing. The results of these experiments are still in the research laboratories, but they give some encouragement to a new approach for fighting viruses.

Tremendous advances in our basic understanding of the biology of viruses offers real hope for the control of these tiny enemies of mankind. The development of antiviral vaccines and drugs for treatment are important not only for the immediate prevention of illness but also for the long-term consequences of viral infection. The role of viruses in producing abnormalities at birth and their possible role in human malignancy puts a high premium on the control of man's smallest and most lethal foes.

The future outlook for the control and prevention of human misery due to viruses undoubtedly will come from advances in the field of molecular biology. Viruses, because of their relatively simple structure and available means of manipulating them in the laboratory, will provide the primary approach to further understanding of the very basis of life. Further knowledge of the enzymes involved in the reproduction of viruses may lead to direct means of prevention or attack. Discovery of hidden or latent viruses which are living in the human body might provide the clues to understanding degenerative diseases and the long-sought-for causes of cancer.

# 20 Some Historical Notes on Coughs and Colds

> The Chincough [whooping cough] generally begins like a common cold, attended with more or less fever. The lips appear full, some degree of hoarseness and sneezing succeed, with a redness or turgescence of the face and generally a watery, irritating discharge from the eyes and nostrils. This febrile state which attends the commencement of Chincough resembles in many respects the fever which precedes the measles or the smallpox.*

Dr. Robert Watt's four children were affected with Chincough, and the two eldest died. Because of the almost total lack of knowledge regarding Chincough, Dr. Watt decided to have his son and daughter examined postmortem in order to learn more about the nature of the disease. He recorded the history of his two children and the findings at autopsy in a book published in 1813. In the appendix to his book, he discusses the morality statistics as a result of the introduction of cowpox vaccination. It

* Robert Watt (see Selected References, p. 163)

was the great hope that the mortality in children would be sharply reduced; as far as the city of Glasgow was concerned, this was not the case. It appears from the registers of deaths that measles became ten times more fatal within the few years that smallpox was being reduced as a result of the introduction of the vaccine.

In Britain, the disease was called Hooping Cough, or the Kink Cough. The "whoop" is the peculiar sound that occurs at the end of a spasm of coughing, as a result of drawing in the breath. The term "Kink cough" is mostly confined to Scotland, and the word "kink" apparently refers to a paroxysm or spasm of coughing. The term was used in connection with laughing or crying, as "a kink (or fit) of laughing." The word "pertussis" dates from Sydenham (1624–89) and is the medical term most commonly employed today for whooping cough.

One of the earliest descriptions of the Chincough was made by Thomas Willis, who practiced first in Oxford and afterward in London and died in 1675. Willis designated the disease as epidemic in nature, occurring commonly in the spring and autumn. The main methods of treatment he recommended were bleeding, vomiting, purging, and blistering. Rosenstein stated that in Sweden, "in the year 1755, 5832 children were carried off by this distemper." In the early 1800's in Glasgow, next to the smallpox and the measles, Chincough was the most fatal disease to which children were liable. Dr. Watt states that the disease is highly contagious, and he cautions: "The universal belief that the system, during the operation of *Pertussis*, generates a specific *virus* capable of communicating the disease, seems to have prevented the mind from looking any farther for a principle adequate to its production." According to Dr. Cullen, "this disease is commonly epidemic and manifestly contagious." "Chincough," says Dr. Hillary, "from all the observations I have been able to make, seems to be equally infectious to children as either the smallpox or measles."

The high susceptibility and predisposition of the newborn was remarked on by Dr. Hamilton. On the mortality in Scotland, Dr. Watt states that only three died in Glasgow above ten years of age out of nearly 2,000. By far the greatest number of deaths occur under the age of two.

"When the kinks are of the Hooping kind, the face as I have already remarked, becomes swollen and of a dark purple color. The veins of the head and neck are extended as if ready to burst and the patient gasps and has the appearance of sudden suffocation. If he remains long in this situation without making any noise, he is said to have taken a *dumb-kink*." *

Dr. Butter records the case of a 30-year-old woman, the mother of several children, who at the time of her Chincough was in a state of pregnancy. A severe fit of coughing was always attended with a clear ropy expectoration. She complained also of pain in her right side, which sometimes shot through to the other, and sometimes downward so as to imitate labor pains. The disease was subdued in a short time by the use of hemlock and other remedies. The patient was afterwards delivered of a healthy child, and had a good recovery."

* Robert Watt (see Selected References, p. 163)

Dr. Watt states further that fever is often very slight and generally subsides as the kinks begin to form. After they are fully formed, it has been imagined that it wholly disappears; hence, Chincough has seldom been ranked among febrile diseases. Sydenham speaks of it as unconnected with fever, and in this sentiment he has been followed by many of our first practitioners. A Chincough is sometimes completely interrupted by the coming on of some other diseases. The following very interesting case is given by Dr. Ferriar of Manchester.

Miss Smith, "aged one year had the Hooping Cough in a slight degree for some weeks. When it seemed to be leaving her, she was seized with the measles and there was the appearance of a very large crop of the eruption. Her cough was not very troublesome and no longer resembled the Hooping Cough. On the third day, she was seized with an extreme degree of dyspnoea, shortness of breath, and a short harrassing cough and the eruption almost entirely disappeared; blisters were applied to different parts of the body; and every method was used to renew the eruption, but without success. The cough increased, but the dyspnoea began to relax, and at length, to my great satisfaction, the type of the Hooping Cough was renewed and my patient recovered by time and change of air."

Dr. Watt states that the history of the Chincough is hardly worth discussing, as most earlier accounts are so exceedingly fanciful and so enveloped in the pathological mist and jargon of former times, that "I have determined to confine this part of the subject within very narrow limits." This might be apropos today, but note what he has to say about the methods of treatment accepted in *his* time. Speaking of purging, he remarks that, "such gentle and gradual evacuations effect the cure as I imagine by easing the lungs, which though they are not found in this distemper to contain much of any serious humour, yet are forced into their violent fits of coughing by fervid and spirituous vapors thrown upon them at certain times by the mass of blood; and are, therefore, best relieved by directing those vapors through the lower bowels and breaking their force by the contrary direction."

The confused state of the leading physicians of that day is probably expressed by the following quotation about the source of the cough. "By some it is placed in the air vessels of the lungs, by others in the alimentary canal, some place it in the superior parts of the air vessels, others in their more minute ramifications, some place it in the pharynx, others in the stomach, and others in the intestines." Dr. Watt believes that the answer will come through dissection and study of the pathological findings. Most pathologists who carried out dissections agree that these patients were suffering from infection of the bronchial tree. Dr. Watt concludes that "signs of neumonic inflammation were very obvious and required the most vigorous means to counterattack them, but it was not until the case of my son occurred that my attention was so strongly directed to the state of the organs of respiration."

His first case is that of his son, Robert Watt, aged six years. He describes his early infancy as being quite normal; that he was a strong, well-developed boy. "About the middle of December he was seized with the symptoms of a *common cold* [Italics mine—J.M.A.] and by Christmas, it appeared pretty obvious that he had gotten the Chin-cough. By the New Year, this was certain, but the symptoms were mild and the only remedies resorted to were an occasional purgative to clear the bowels. As soon as the kinks were formed, he vomited freely, particularly after meals. He had also occasionally some bleeding from the nose and though he sometimes looked a little paler than usual, we discovered no remarkable abatement either in his health or spirits. After New Year's the kinks became more severe and were accompanied by a profuse expectoration of a very tough mucus. The vomitting continued, but he ate some of his meals heartily. We were now disposed to take him from school, but from the fear of being left behind by his companions, he was exceedingly averse to the measure and therefore continued to attend regularly until Friday, the 8th of January. On this evening he had some calomel combined with a little tartarised antimony, which operated powerfully both as an emetic and purgative. The next day, his breathing was harder and his pulse was quicker, but he still appeared to be in good spirits as usual. At bedtime, he took two aloetic pills, which operated next morning.

"On the following day because of breathlessness, a large blister was applied to the breast. A shortness of breath and rapid pulse continued. Further purging was done without results and bleeding was resorted to. About five ounces of blood were taken from his arm. About 4 o'clock on the morning of Tuesday, he was so exceedingly distressed that bleeding was again resolved on, and from 5 to 6 ounces were taken from the jugular. The relief obtained from this operation was less obvious, and more transitory, than from the former."

Further treatment followed: "A blister was also applied to the chest, and several attempts were made to procure an evacuation from the bowels, he was also put into the warm bath; but the return of night, showed that all was unavailing. On Wednesday, about four ounces were taken from the back of one of his hands and an emetic was again administered on the advice of a friend. Early on the morning of Thursday, he appeared at times to be delirious. Part of his head was shaven, and a blister applied. A large blister was applied to the under part of the chest and upper part of the abdomen. Every other attempt to relieve him having failed, it was now resolved to try the effect of wine."

A further quotation reads as follows: "At each kink, he rose, with a little assistance to his hands and knees, with his head over the bedside. He continued to do this until about 7 in the evening when he made the usual demonstrations, by throwing down the bedclothes off his body but, as if he had forgotten what he was going to do, he lay still, had a sort of weaker kink than usual, and in a few minutes breathed his last without the smallest struggle. His death from what was discovered on dissection appeared to have been occasioned by the entire plugging up of the air cells and bronchi with fluid."

Dr. Watt describes the second case, that of his daughter, Janet Watt, aged four and a half years. The details of her illness will not be recorded here. In both of the two cases the surface of the lungs was irregularly covered with whitish spots slightly elevated. "On speaking of this circumstance to my late worthy and much respected friend, Mr. Allen Burns, he mentioned that it was not a very uncommon appearance—he had met with it often. 'It seemed,' he remarked, 'to be always connected with an inflamed state of the lungs themselves or of the passages leading to them.' "

# 21 Epilogue

*I AM AT THIS MOMENT*
*DEAF IN THE EARS,*
*HOARSE IN THE THROAT,*
*RED IN THE NOSE,*
*GREEN IN THE GILLS,*
*DAMP IN THE EYES,*
*TWITCHY IN THE JOINTS,*
*AND FRACTIOUS IN TEMPER*
*FROM A MOST INTOLERABLE*
*AND OPPRESSIVE COLD.*[*]

—Charles Dickens

A cold may be defined as a contagious minor illness with running nose, stuffiness, scratchy throat, cough, and little

[*] From the presidential address delivered by Dr. John H. Dingle before the American Association of Immunologists, Philadelphia, Pennsylvania, April 15, 1958. In *The Collected Letters of Charles Dickens,* Vol. I, p. 92 (London: Chapman and Hall Ltd., 1880).

or no fever. Fortunately, these mild symptoms account for the great majority of what people call "colds," but the story does not end here. The cause of colds is now known: most of them are caused by newly discovered viruses. They bounce from nose to nose after we sneeze, cough, and talk. Many of them do not cause any symptoms but infect us and produce antibodies, which protect against the particular virus invading again, for a while at least. These same viruses are not always so kind and gentle, but proceed to cause more severe symptoms, such as croup, hoarseness, earaches, and signs of bronchitis and pneumonia. Some cause acute inflammation of the heart, and in babies this complication is frequently fatal. On occasion these *same* viruses which cause the mild trivial illnesses may produce headache and drowsiness, with high fever, convulsions, and inflammation of the brain.

A large group of viruses known as rhinoviruses recently discovered in England and the United States is a very common cause of colds in adults. In infants and children, other viruses seem to cause most of the acute respiratory illnesses. These are known as "croup agents," adenoviruses, and respiratory syncytial virus. The latter is considered the commonest cause of pneumonia in infants, but may cause minor illness in human volunteers and adults. Many of the respiratory viruses cause a coldlike illness when tested in human adult volunteers. The polioviruses and those closely related to them cause "summer colds," and that may be all there is to it; but they may on *rare* occasions cause paralysis and death. Polio vaccines are safe and effective and should be given to everyone.

Influenza is a world-wide disease and may attack infants, children, and adults alike. The disease is mild for the most part, but each epidemic leaves a wake of death following its periodic visits. The newer vaccines have been found to protect 60 to 80 per cent of persons who are fully immunized.

The symptoms of common measles, cough, running nose, and mild inflammation in the eyes, are like a cold. These are followed by a rash, and this may be all, with prompt recovery and immunity for life. Several hundred children die annually in the United States as a result of measles; thousands die in India; and it is the commonest cause of death in children in some countries in Africa. The virus of measles may cause pneumonia or may be mixed with bacteria to cause serious complications. The most serious complication is measles encephalitis and its aftereffects. It may cause brain damage in half of the individuals affected. The new measles vaccines are safe and effective and should be given to everyone who has not had regular measles.

The cause of "sudden unexpected death" in infants is not known. It has been shown, however, that most of these tragic events are related to signs of inflammation in the respiratory passages. The baby's first experience with common viruses (when he has lost the protection of the antibodies from his mother) may be a serious, overwhelming, fatal illness.

Viruses are tiny living organisms composed of complicated chemical molecules known as deoxyribonucleic acid, DNA, and ribonucleic acid, RNA. The mechanism by which they reproduce themselves is now revealed, and thus through viruses, the simplest living forms, we are actually learning about the "secret of life" itself. They may be stopped in the process of reproduction by substances which interfere with the way they operate. One of these substances which stops viruses is interferon. It is made by cells when they are attacked by viruses and probably is the main reason why recovery from the initial illness takes place so promptly. It is still not available to treat disease, but it represents a great advance in our basic understanding of these common illnesses. The common antibiotics have no direct effect on viruses and are *not* indicated in the treatment of most of these uncomplicated infections. A wise choice of drugs may be made when your doctor has evidence of a complicating infection.

Emphasis in this book has been placed on the *causes* of illness rather than on the area of the body that may be affected. There are dozens of causes of tonsillitis or sore throat. By means of careful history, thorough examination of the patient, a knowledge of incidence (what diseases are prevalent and in what seasons), plus the aid of laboratory tests if indicated, a practical working diagnosis can usually be made. It is important to know the probable cause of the illness in determining the best treatment. The illness could be influenza, mumps, measles, Coxsackie, tuberculosis, or a "strep" infection. Wiser treatment will result from a conscientious effort to arrive at an accurate diagnosis. This is not always easy, but it would seem to be the most logical and sensible approach to the problem. Unfortunately the ordinary antibiotics are rarely the answer in the management of acute respiratory illnesses. *Rest* and *good nursing care,* with a close watch for complications, are the main principles to follow.

Hopefully, the day will come when O. Henry's definition of life will not be true. Life will not be "made up of sobs, sniffles and smiles, with sniffles predominating."

# Glossary

*Antibodies:* Substances produced by cells in response to stimulating agents such as viruses or bacteria. They are quite *specific* in their ability to protect against infection—that is, polio antibodies will protect against poliomyelitis only.

*Bacteria:* Plural for bacterium, which is a general term for a *germ* such as the tubercle bacillus (which causes tuberculosis) or streptococcus (which may cause sore throats and scarlet fever).

*Bronchiolitis:* Inflammation of the smallest tubes in the lung, which extend between the larger bronchi and the air sacs. It is really bronchopneumonia.

*Carditis:* Inflammation of the heart, which may be caused by viruses or bacteria and rarely other agents.

*Cell:* The body is made up almost entirely of many different kinds of cells. Each cell has a discrete inner core, which is called the *nucleus,* surrounded by material called *cytoplasm.* The cell is encased in a membrane separating it from other cells.

*Clinical:* Pertaining to the actual observation and treatment of *patients,* as distinguished from theoretical or experimental observations.

*Conjunctivitis:* Inflammation of the eyes, as "pink eye."

*Coryza:* A "cold" in the head, running nose. Allergic coryza is hay fever or rhinitis.

*Deoxyribonucleic Acid* (DNA): The chemical substance in the core or nucleus of the cell or virus. It is the molecules that contain the genetic code and determine the pattern of the offspring.

*Diagnosis:* The art of distinguishing one disease from another.

*Differential Diagnosis:* The determination of which one of two or more diseases a patient is suffering from by systematically comparing the findings.

*Enanthem:* A rash or spots *inside* the mouth or throat.

*Encephalitis:* Inflammation of the brain, sometimes called "sleeping sickness," caused by viruses and other microscopic organisms.

*Enzymes:* Compounds, frequently proteins, capable of producing a chemical reaction.

*Eosinophils:* White blood cells sometimes found in increased numbers in allergic conditions.

*Epidemiology:* The science concerned with the cause, frequency, and distribution of infectious diseases.

*Etiology:* The study of the *causes* of diseases.

*Exanthem:* A rash on the *outside* of the body or on the skin.

*Exudate:* A substance, often forming a whitish membrane or spots in the throat or on the tonsils.

*Fungus:* Any one of a class of vegetable organisms of a low order, as molds or yeast.

*Gamma Globulin:* A protein fraction of the blood serum, which is known to contain many different kinds of antibodies.

*Hepatitis:* Inflammation of the liver.

*Incubation period:* The time between the exposure to the causative agent and the beginning of symptoms.

*Interferon:* An interfering substance that neutralizes viruses. It is produced by the body's cells in response to foreign nucleic acid, such as viruses. It protects uninfected cells.

*Laryngitis:* Inflammation of the voice box; hoarseness and "croup" are symptoms of laryngitis.

*Malignancy:* A cancerous process which spreads from the site of origin.

*Mycoplasma:* Smallest germs capable of growth in a culture medium without cells.

*Nephritis:* Inflammation of the kidney.

*Nucleotide:* A compound which results from the splitting of nucleic acid by the enzyme nuclease.

*Pharyngitis:* Inflammation of the throat.

*Prognosis:* A forecast as to the probable result of an attack of disease; or, prospects for recovery.

*Rhinitis:* Coryza or running nose.

*Ribonucleic Acid* (RNA): The chemical substance that transfers or carries the pattern to the protein factories in the cell. Some viruses are made up of RNA.

*Rickettsia:* Microscopic organisms that are intermediate between bacteria and viruses; often transmitted by ticks.

*Rubella:* A disease with a measly-like rash, often called "three-day measles" or German measles, due to rubella virus. It is not measles.

*Rubeola:* Regular or common measles with blotchy rash, cough, running nose, and inflamed eyes, due to rubeola virus.

*Sequela:* A condition following or caused by a previous disease; an aftereffect of illness.

*Stool:* Excreta from the lower bowel, or "bowel movement."

*Tissue culture:* Living tissue cells growing in special solutions conducive to their growth, usually in glass tubes or bottles.

*Titer:* A level, or *strength* of a substance such as antibodies in serum.

*Virus:* A living agent, the smallest and simplest form of life, which depends on other living cells in order to replicate or reproduce itself. From the *Oxford English Dictionary,* 1778: "Venice is a stink-pot, charged with the very virus of hell!" Prior to the ending of the nineteenth century, *virus* was known as a foul, offensive, poisonous fluid. In 1892, Iwanowski, a Russian, first reported the results of filtration experiments (keeping out bacteria) with tobacco-mosaic disease. Independently, a Dutchman, Beijerinck, in 1898 repeated the same experiments. He realized that a new type of infectious agent, which he called *contagium vivum fluidum,* had been discovered.

# Selected References


Adams, J. M. (1960): Newer Virus Diseases: Clinical Differentiation of Acute Respiratory Infections. The Macmillan Company, New York.

Adams, J. M. (1964): Acute Respiratory Diseases. Brennemann-Kelley Practice of Pediatrics, Vol. II, Chapter 40.

Adams, J. M. (1964): Recent Advances in Pediatrics. Presented by invitation at the 120th Annual Meeting of The American Psychiatric Association. Am. J. of Psych., 121:572.

Adams, J. M. (1966): Etiologic and Clinical Aspects of Acute Respiratory Disease in Children. Advances in Cardiopulmonary Diseases. Year Book Medical Publishers, Chicago, Illinois, Vol. III, p. 166.

Adams, J. M., D. T. Imagawa, and K. Zike (1961): Epidemic Bronchiolitis and Pneumonitis Related to Respiratory Syncytial Virus. J. of the Amer. Med. Assoc., 176:1037–1039.

Adams, J. M., and N. Smith (1946): Clinical Trial of Gamma Globulin in the Prevention of Common Respiratory Diseases. Proc. Soc. Exper. Biol. and Med., 63:446.

Andrewes, C. H. (1964): The Complex Epidemiology of Respiratory Virus Infections. Science, 146:1274.

Andrewes, C. H. (1965): The Common Cold. Weidenfeld and Nicolson, London.

Andrewes, C. H. (1965): The Troubles of a Virus. J. Gen. Microbiol., 40:149–156.

Babb, J. M., M. E. R. Stoneman, and H. Stern (1961): Myocarditis and Croup Caused by Coxsackie Virus Type B5. Archives of Dis. in Childhood, 36:551–556.

Bakwin, H. (1958): The Tonsil-Adenoidectomy Enigma. J. Pediat., 52:339.

Breese, B. B. (1962): Clinical Conference: Diagnosis and Treatment of Streptococcal Infections in Children. Pediatric Conference from The Babies' Hospital Unit, United Hospitals of Newark, New Jersey, 5:1–12.

Burnet, Sir Macfarlane (1962): Natural History of Infectious Disease. The Syndics of the Cambridge University Press, New York.

Chanock, R. M., and R. H. Parrott (1965): Acute Respiratory Disease in Infancy and Childhood. Pediatrics, 36:21–39.

Chanock, R. M., et al. (1966): Immunization by Selective Infection with Type 4 Adenovirus Grown in Human Diploid Tissue Culture. J.A.M.A., 195:445–459.

Conference on Newer Respiratory Disease Viruses, Bethesda, Maryland, October 3, 4, 5 (1962): The American Review of Respiratory Diseases, 88:1–419, September, 1963.

Current Virus Research (1959): British Medical Bulletin, Vol. 15.

Delaney, T. B. and F. H. Fukanago (1958): Myocarditis in a Newborn Infant with Encephalomeningitis due to Coxsackie Virus Group B, Type 4. New England J. of Med., 259:234–236.

Dewhurst, K. (1964): Thomas Willis as a Physician. University of California, Los Angeles.

Diehl, H. S., A. B. Baker, and D. W. Cowan (1938): Cold Vaccines, An Evaluation Based on a Controlled Study. J.A.M.A., 111:1168.

Dingle, J. H. (1960): Certain Clinical and Climatological Characteristics of the Common Cold. Transactions of the American Clinical and Climatological Association, 72:18.

Dingle, J. H. (1958): The Curious Case of the Common Cold. J. of Immunology, 81:91–97.

Fabricant, N. D., and G. Conklin (1965): The Dangerous Cold. The Macmillan Company, New York.

Glaser, J. (1956): Allergy in Childhood. Charles C Thomas, Springfield, Illinois.

Hamparian, V. V., M. B. Leagus, and M. R. Hilleman (1964): Additional Rhinovirus Serotypes. Proc. Soc. Exper. Biol. and Med., 116:976–984.

Hilleman, M. R. (1963): Respiratory Viruses and Respiratory Virus Vaccines. Am. Review of Respiratory Diseases, 87:165–180.

Hilleman, M. R. (1964): Prospects for the Role of Viruses in Human Malignancy. Health Laboratory Science, Vol. 1.

Isaacs, A., and J. Lindenmann: Virus Interference. I. The Interferon. Proc. Roy. Soc. B., 1957, V147, 258–267.

Jackson, G. G., H. F. Dowling, L. W. Akers, R. L. Muldoon, A. Van Dyke, and G. C. Johnson (1962): Immunity to the Common Cold from Protective Serum Antibody: Time of Appearance, Persistence and Relation to Re-infection. New England J. of Med., 266:791–796.

Jansson, E., O. Wager, P. Forssel, and H. Halonen (1961): An Exanthema Subitum-like Rash in Patients with Adenovirus Infection. Annales Pediatrica Fenn., Vol. 7.

Katz, S. L. (1964): Efficacy, Potential and Hazards of Vaccines. New England J. of Med., 270:884–889.

Komrower, G. M., B. L. Williams, and P. B. Stones (1955): Lymphocytic Choriomeningitis in the Newborn: Probably Transplacental Infection. Lancet, pp. 697–698.

Lennette E. H., R. L. Magoffin, W. A. Longshore, Jr., and A. C. Hollister, Jr. (1961): An Etiologic Study of Seasonal Aseptic Meningitis and Encephalitis in the Central Valley of California. Am. J. of Tropical Med. and Hygiene, 10:885–896.

Lewis, J. M., and J. P. Utz (1961): Orchitis, Parotitis and Meningoencephalitis Due to Lymphocytic-Choriomeningitis Virus. New England J. of Med., 265:776–780.

Miller, W. S. (1937): The Lung. Charles C Thomas, Springfield, Illinois.

Mufson, M. S., M. A. Manko, J. R. Kingston, and R. M. Chanock (1961): Eaton Agent Pneumonia—Clinical Features. J. of the Amer. Med. Assoc., 178:369–374.

Oseasohn, R. (1963): The Use of Family Groups in the Study of Respiratory Disease. The American Review of Respiratory Diseases, 88:110.

Panum, Peter Ludwig: Observations Made During the Epidemic of Measles on the Faroe Islands in the Year 1846. Medical Classics, May, 1939, Vol. 3.

Phaire, Thomas (1965): The Boke of Chyldren. E. & S. Livingstone, Ltd., Edinburgh and London (First published in 1553).

Portnoy, B. and P. F. Wehrle (1963): Respiratory Diseases of Viral Etiology. Current Concepts in Chest Diseases, Vol. III.

Report of the Committee on the Control of Infectious Diseases (1964): American Academy of Pediatrics.

Sabin, A. B. (1965): Contribution of Virology to Human Medicine during the Past 40 Years. Israel J. Med. Sc., 6:1090–1098.

Sanders, V. (1963): Viral Myocarditis. Am. Heart J., St. Louis, 66:707–713.

Schmidt, N. J. (1964): Trends in the Laboratory Diagnosis of Viral Infections. Postgraduate Medicine, 35:488.

Smith, K. M. (1964): Viruses. Cambridge University Press.

Smith, W. (1963): Mechanisms of Virus Infection. Academic Press. London and New York.

Sussman, M. S., L. Strauss, and H. L. Hodes (1959): Fatal Coxsackie Group B Virus Infection in the Newborn: Report of a Case with Necroscopy Findings and Brief Review of the Literature. A.M.A. J. Dis. Childhood, 97:483–492.

Tamm, I., and H. J. Eggers (1963): Specific Inhibition of Replication of Animal Viruses. Science, 142:24.

University of California: Radio-Television Broadcast (1963): The Thread of Life. Broadcast #6047-U.E. 1837.

Utz, J. P., and A. I. Shelokov (1958): Coxsackie B Virus Infection: Presence of Virus in Blood, Urine, and Cerebrospinal Fluid. J. of the Amer. Med. Assoc., Vol. 168.

van Creveld, S., and J. De Jager (1965): Myocarditis in Newborns, Caused by Coxsackie Virus. Clinical and Pathological Data. International Review of Pediat., 187: 101–112.

Walker, S. H., and Y. Togo (1963): Encephalitis Due to Group B,

Type 5 Coxsackie Virus. Am. J. of Dis. of Child., 105:209–212.

Walters, J. H. (1960): Postencephalitic Parkinson Syndrome After Meningo-encephalitis due to Coxsackie Virus Group B, Type 2. New England J. of Med., 263:744–747.

Watt, Robert (1813): The History, Nature and Treatment of Chincough. John Smith and Son, London.

Wheatley, G. M. (1963): Respiratory Disease in Children. Bulletin of the National Tuberculosis Association, March.

Wilkins, M. H. F. (1963): Molecular Configuration of Nucleic Acids. Science, 140:941.

Williams, Greer (1960): Virus Hunters. Alfred A. Knopf, New York.

Zinsser, Hans (1935): Rats, Lice and History. George Routledge & Sons, Ltd., London.

# Index

Numbers in **boldface type** indicate primary discussion of the topic.